Clinics in Developmental Medicine No. 161
MANAGEMENT OF THE MOTOR
DISORDERS OF CHILDREN WITH
CEREBRAL PALSY. 2ND EDITION

Senior Editor: Martin C.O. Bax
Editor: Hilary M. Hart
Managing Editor: Michael Pountney
Sub Editor: Pat Chappelle

First published in this edition 2004

British Library Cataloguing-in-Publication data:
A catalogue record for this book is available from the British Library

ISSN: 0069 4835
ISBN: 1 898683 32 8

Printed by The Lavenham Press Ltd, Water Street, Lavenham, Suffolk
Mac Keith Press is supported by Scope

**Books are to be returned on or before
the last date below.**

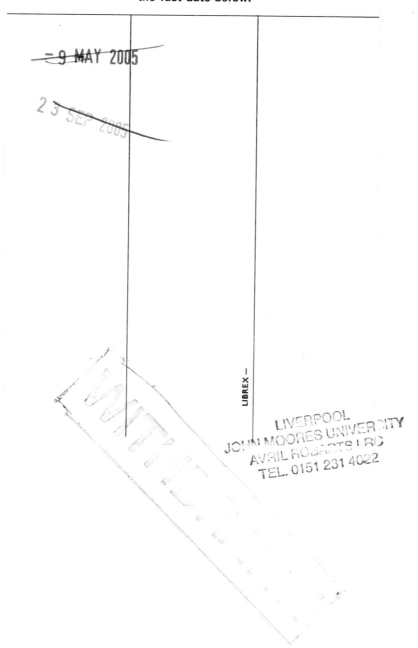

= 9 MAY 2005

2 3 SEP 2005

LIBREX —

LIVERPOOL
JOHN MOORES UNIVERSITY
AVRIL ROBARTS LRC
TEL. 0151 231 4022

Clinics in Developmental Medicine No. 161

Management of the Motor Disorders of Children with Cerebral Palsy

2nd Edition

Edited by

DAVID SCRUTTON
Institute of Child Health
University College London
England

DIANE DAMIANO
Washington University
St Louis, MO, USA

MARGARET MAYSTON
Department of Physiology
University College London
England

2004
Mac Keith Press

Distributed by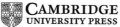

CONTENTS

ACKNOWLEDGEMENT

The editors would like to thank Martin Bax not only for his insistent reminders that a second edition was needed, but also for his tactful suggestion that the subject now demanded a radical departure from the first edition.

AUTHORS' APPOINTMENTS

Martin Bax

Emeritus Reader in Paediatrics, Imperial College of Medicine, Department of Child Health, Chelsea and Westminster Hospital, London, England

Eva Bower

Senior Lecturer, School of Health Professions and Rehabilitation Sciences, University of Southampton, England

Roslyn N. Boyd

Senior Research Physiotherapist, Neonatal Neurology, Murdoch Children's Research Institute; *and* Senior Lecturer, School of Physiotherapy, La Trobe University, Melbourne, Victoria, Australia

J. Keith Brown

Consultant Paediatric Neurologist, Royal Hospital for Sick Children, Edinburgh, Scotland

Diane Damiano

Research Associate Professor of Neurology; Adjunct Associate Professor of Physical Therapy; *and* Director, Shared Movement Assessment Center, Washington University, St Louis, MO, USA

Susan Edwards

Clinical Specialist Physiotherapist, Stoke Mandeville Hospital and Bobath Centre, London, England

Mary Galea

Professor of Clinical Physiotherapy, School of Physiotherapy, University of Melbourne, Parkville, Victoria, Australia

Murray Goldstein

Chief Operating Officer and Medical Director, UCP Research and Educational Foundation, Washington DC, USA

H. Kerr Graham	Professor of Orthopaedic Surgery, University of Melbourne; Director of Orthopaedic Surgery, Royal Children's Hospital; and Director, Hugh Williamson Gait Analysis Laboratory, Royal Children's Hospital, Melbourne, Victoria, Australia
Jean-Pierre Lin	Consultant Paediatric Neurologist, Guy's and St Thomas' NHS Trust, London, England
Margaret Mayston	Lecturer, Department of Physiology, University College London, England
Sheila McNeill	Senior I Paediatric Physiotherapist, Mitchell House and Fleming Fulton Schools, Green Park Healthcare Trust, Belfast, Northern Ireland
Peter Rosenbaum	Professor of Paediatrics, Canada Research Chair in Childhood Disability, and Co-Director, *CanChild* Centre for Childhood Disability Research, McMaster University, Hamilton, Ontario, Canada
David Scrutton	Honorary Senior Lecturer, Institute of Child Health, University College London, and Guy's, King's College and St Thomas' Hospitals, King's College, London, England

FOREWORD

The first edition of this book was a welcome introduction to the most commonly used systems and treatment philosophies for cerebral palsy as they were perceived nearly 20 years ago. It is still useful as an introduction, but knowledge and societal attitudes have changed and a revision was needed. For this new edition the editors bring together outstanding individuals who have contributed new knowledge and a wealth of experience to this field, to provide perspective on current thinking in the treatment of cerebral palsy.

Cerebral palsy is an important common disorder that children experience and adapt to as they grow and develop into adults. It is a lifelong condition that challenges the individual child, their family and ultimately the individual as an adult. Society is also challenged, as are the health professionals who seek to understand the disorder and to develop effective interventions that reduce the primary and secondary consequences. We need to face up to the challenge of integrating our current knowledge and stimulating our drive to develop new knowledge.

Children's health professionals, particularly those working with chronic disability, view themselves as part of an interdisciplinary group, each relying on the experience and expertise of others in the team. Most of us have always seen parents as the key to the child's success but increasingly this is being more strongly emphasized. We all need truly to engage parents within a therapeutic environment and appreciate that the way we organize and deliver care and work with families has an impact on outcomes, both in the short term and in the longer term.

The advancement in our practice is dependent on many factors, not least being increasing our understanding of specific etiologies and their natural histories, for without a picture of the child's more likely future it is hard to establish the priorities of any intervention. We need to have an understanding of how the body grows and the changes that occur in cerebral palsy which lead to deformity, and how we might prevent, ameliorate or correct them; how children learn to move, and how (and how much) we can influence this process to the child's advantage; and how and to what extent environmental factors can influence the natural history of the disorder.

We have made progress. The last decade has seen the development of a range of new interventions for management of children with cerebral palsy and these face the clinician with a more complex set of decisions to make when assessing any particular child. Therapeutic interventions now cover an ever greater field of expertise: general care, oral medications, intrathecal medications, selective dorsal rhizotomy, botulinum toxin A, muscle strengthening, seating and positioning, serial casting and orthotics, life styles and a broad range of physiotherapy approaches.

However, underpinning this evolution of therapeutics has been the increasing expectation for evidence-based decision making which has been driven in part by the development of the means of accurately measuring treatment effect. There is still a long way to go, and in spite of the advances in our knowledge all too often we still rely on 'clinical experience' as the principle source of information related to effective interventions.

As our field of childhood expertise matures we become increasingly aware of the issues related to adults who have cerebral palsy. Surprisingly little attention has been paid to this area and its inclusion in this book is both appropriate and timely.

The editors have brought together key experts in the field of cerebral palsy across multiple disciplines to give readers a practical and current view of what we know and where we need to go in the future. I think this will be an important reference for the practicing clinician to use in their day-to-day work with children, youths and adults with cerebral palsy.

Bob Armstrong
President, American Academy of Cerebral Palsy and Developmental Medicine
January 2004

1
INTRODUCTION

David Scrutton

In the first edition of this book, I set out to persuade the proponents of the current and generally accepted methods of treatment in cerebral palsy (CP) to write about their treatments. Each author was asked to follow a chapter structure outlining the aims, rationale and methods of their particular treatment. The purpose was to remove some of the confusion and mystique that most non-therapists (and not a few therapists) found when trying to discover what the physical treatment of these children was all about. However, attitudes to these treatments have moved on, and today that rather didactic and divisive approach is inappropriate and outdated. It has been said that people are either 'splitters' or 'joiners', and in that sense perhaps the first book was to help the former and this edition is to encourage the latter.

Since Jennie Colby at the end of the 19th century (Slominski 1984) separated the therapy (such as it was) for children with cerebral motor disorders and good intellect from those with severe developmental delay, fresh ideas have flowed and ebbed, some leaving behind an idea that was absorbed into the generally accepted management of these children. The first edition was fortunate in that it was published at a time when the debate about which treatment method was best was at its height, and this allowed a representative cross section of views to be expressed. Such discussion continues to this day and will go on until there is sufficient research to show us what is correct (see Chapters 4, 5). As fresh ideas and, more importantly, knowledge have crept in, most arguments have quietly slipped into history, and a few once-novel treatment methods have become accepted practice. However, established practices do not disappear overnight, and some treatments have survived by assimilating modern practice into their ambit to the extent that they no longer truly represent what they continue to propound (see Chapter 10). Pretending to be different and in some way 'special', they actually treat using selected parts only of the common pool of modalities, masking the reality behind their jargon.

The days of those preaching their 'one true modality' have gone. Instead of certainty we have search; and therapy is evolving. That change has been accompanied by another and greater change. Those of us who considered that the family is the key to success or failure of treatment for CP once faced a professional environment that saw anything outside the treatment room as 'good' but 'second best'. I think that too has passed into history (see Chapter 3). It is now generally acknowledged that the efficacy of any physical treatment lies within the child's day-to-day environment, and to pretend otherwise is a professional conceit. As long ago as the 1940s Eirene Collis understood this, but even she with all her aggressive holism couldn't quite bring herself to write it and give away so much professional 'power' (Collis 1947). Thirty years ago I was asked at a meeting what was the most important thing I looked for in a therapist when interviewing and I replied, "Humility". It was not seen as a good answer. Humility is still needed but it is now more readily available.

So the needs met by the first edition hardly exist today and a new edition has become essential. Change implied that it be edited by those at the forefront of current practice, and the aim was to have a combination of nationalities and wide knowledge of clinical, academic and research experience in the physical treatment of these children. The need has been fully met through the efforts of Diane Damiano (from the USA) and Margaret Mayston (from Australia, currently working in the UK). Together we decided that we should not attempt to update the first edition, which can stand on its own as a reference for *temps perdu*, but that instead a completely different book should be planned.

This is not a book explaining *how* to treat CP; rather, it explains to therapists, doctors, teachers, carers and parents *why* we do what we do, *how* we think about it and what may be possible *in the future*. It aims to offer something for all the children's upbringing and physical management (see

What is going on during 'treatment'?

Watching a therapist treat a child often raises questions. What are they doing? To what end? How often do they need to do it? When will the difference be apparent? What may not be immediately obvious is that many less experienced therapists are a bit puzzled too, and many are treating with a nagging feeling that there are 'better' treatments than theirs, going on 'somewhere' (Scrutton 2000). This is because some of those who lecture about treatment do so in exaggerated terms that imply (and a few clearly claim) how very effective the treatment is; and therapists with little experience believe them (for what professional does not wish to be more effective?). When they cannot match their expectations they tend at first to blame their incompetence rather than the over-sell. Some 'named' therapies are blatant in their claims, and the same can be said, for instance, of some quite simple treatment techniques and novel orthotic designs.

Very few of the treatments for CP have been fully researched. The majority of conventional practice is founded either upon 'common sense' (for example: children are more comfortable and can use their hands better in chairs that fit their needs) or upon clinical observations that have stood the test of time. In the first edition I attempted to look at treatment from the point of view of defining aims and wrote about it under the title of 'aim-oriented' treatment. In retrospect I think this may have been mistaken as everyone who treats thinks they have an aim (however imprecise or misguided it may be), and the point I was trying to make was that the aims had to be specific and time-precise, rather than 'sitting better' or something similar. So what should the interested observer be looking for when analysing a treatment?

1. How is the Therapy Meant to Influence the Child's Movements?

There is a spectrum of aims that helps to define one aspect of a treatment. At the most radical end of this spectrum are three treatments that claim to be *altering* the structure of the central nervous system (CNS): two only in infancy (Katona and Vojta), and one at any age (Doman). Moving along the spectrum, there are treatments that aim to *train* the CNS. How this differs

2

from 'altering' and exactly what 'training' and 'altering' mean is debatable (see Chapter 6), and these words are used too loosely on occasions. Some of these treatments aim to change *basic movement patterns* (*e.g.* Bobath/NDT), which are then 'available' for any function. Whereas two treatments in particular concentrate on training the individual *functions* (Collis and Conductive Education [CE]), one of these (CE) and most 'conventional' therapy set out to show alternative strategies that are optimal for a particular child to achieve a specific goal. At the far end of the spectrum and merging into these pattern-acquiring and function-training treatments is a style of treatment often called (usually derogatorily) 'traditional' or 'conventional' therapy, implying that the child has a treatment akin to 'exercises' to strengthen weak muscles, stretch tight joints, and practise the use of the upper limbs, correct posture, balance and walking. This latter approach to treatment is rather more immediately understood by most people, because it is what they understand by the words 'physical therapy' and 'exercise'. While 'conventional' treatment is by no means alone in preventing secondary pathology, it does so rather more directly. This is because some of the other treatments see the overall effect of their regimen to produce postures and movements that are not going to cause (say) deformity, whereas 'conventional' therapy aims rather more directly to prevent or correct such secondary pathology.

2. WHAT IS THE MODE OF INTERVENTION?
These can be categorized under three headings:
• *Treatments that act directly upon what is to be changed:* for example, if the knee movement isn't strong enough, treat the muscles acting across the knee joint. If a joint is stiff, move it.
• *Neurophysiological:* treatments based on different aspects of neurological function; utilizing exteroception and proprioception to increase or decrease muscle action and so affect CNS activity. This is rather different from the first mode as the parts of the body being handled are not necessarily the parts intended to be affected.
• *Educational:* creating interactions with the child, which appear to owe more to 'education' than to physical treatment or 'exercises', to encourage better movement and function.

All treatments will have elements of each but one will predominate.

3. HOW TARGETED IS THE TREATMENT?
Some treatments have quite specific and limited aims, *e.g.* methods of relaxing a spastic muscle group or increasing the range of movement at a joint. Other treatments have a more global approach to the disability and take on the role of a philosophy of treatment.

4. WHO DOES THE TREATMENT?
Some treatments require special skills and experience, and although parents or care staff could be shown how to do them, they would be unlikely to be competent enough to achieve as much as a therapist. Other treatments are specifically designed to be done by lay people, their effect being enhanced by constant application rather than diminished through lack of expertise. Whereas it may be obvious that some of the specific treatment techniques require special skills from the therapist, it may not be so apparent that this also applies to the lay

treatments. The formulation of a treatment programme (however simple it might appear) and instruction of parents in its application are not something that anyone can do without guidance or experience.

5. WHAT IS THE PRIMARY AIM?
Some treatments aim for better patterns of movement, greater postural stability and increased joint range, in the expectation that these will automatically expand the child's movement opportunities and so increase function. Other treatments aim directly for function, considering that the abilities and attitudes engendered in the child are of primary importance, and that treatments not so directed do not automatically lead to increased day-to-day competence and may impede other aspects of the child's development. The latter view seems to be gaining the ascendant.

6. WHAT AGE GROUP IS SUITABLE?
The suitability of a treatment can depend on the child's age: a treatment may be inappropriate because it requires either cooperation from the child which cannot be expected without a certain level of maturity; or handling by the therapist which cannot easily be achieved if the child is too large. Equally, the rationale may be based on neurodevelopmental considerations, relying on the 'plasticity' of the as yet uncommitted CNS, aiming to influence the development of new skills prior to or during their emergence. Thus some treatments are suitable only for particular ages or stages of development, while others may be applicable throughout life.

As with any classification these categories cannot be comprehensive; other factors subdivide the treatments. However, they allow a comparison of what is going on that may be of help to readers, particular those not directly involved in treating children with CP.

The best treatment
A question often asked of therapists and paediatricians is "What is the best treatment for cerebral palsy?" There is no generally applicable answer because the 'best' treatment is the one most appropriate for the particular child, their circumstances (family, school, locality) and the facilities and expertise available. The most important thing is to have the correct aims of treatment. It may be better to achieve a little of the most important aim than all of a less important one. Only when the priority of aims has been decided can one begin to ask "How do we achieve them?" (for there will seldom be only one aim or only one way of achieving it). Even then rational judgements often cannot be made because there may be little evidence on what is the best thing to do. It is generally accepted that this lack of evidence is due mainly to the complexity of the condition (see Chapters 2, 7) and that children, unlike adults, are continuously changing with or without treatment. Although research will gradually chip away at our ignorance, it unlikely that a simple model applicable to all will ever emerge.

The uncertainty of very early diagnosis and the imprecision of the prognosis dictates that alterations of outcome through treatment are most likely to be shown only from trials involving large numbers of children. An incidence of approximately two per 1000 live births makes this difficult, so it must involve multicentre trials, which themselves introduce further difficulties. Trials require standardized diagnostic techniques and terminology (which are difficult) and standardized treatments (which are nearly impossible for all but the simplest, *e.g.* plastering a joint at a particular angle for a set time). It seems likely that progress will be made first of all in two areas: assessing specific techniques applied to specific presenting signs secondary to CP (*e.g.* prevention or correction of deformity—see Chapters 8, 9), and the gradual introduction of more reliable and early prognostic tests, probably through greatly refined methods of assessing residual function of the CNS at an early age.

Early treatment

In the meantime, while also advocating the need for treatment of older children or adults, most therapists favour early treatment, and there is general agreement that the younger the child the greater the effect of the treatment. There are a number of reasons why this might be so:

• Massive myelination and pathway selection is occurring and it is probably easier to form correct movement habits before incorrect ones are established.

• Most parents expect to devote a large proportion of their time to a baby during its first two years of life and so it is easier and more realistic for them to involve themselves in consistent treatment.

• Treatment does not interfere with the education and social life of the child.

• It is a time when parents need close contact with someone who understands their problems in a constructive manner, is able to give them something positive to do and can help them to find out about and understand their child's emerging difficulties.

• When treatment does start one of the first questions the parent will ask is, "Would treatment have been more effective if we had started sooner?" It is difficult to answer that question convincingly in any way other than "yes", otherwise the next question is "Then why start now?".

The difficulty in diagnosis and accurate prognosis before the age of 6 months allows the cynical to suggest that it is easier to ameliorate (or even 'cure') a disorder that may not be present than one that is definitely there, and it must be admitted that there is probably a not inconsiderable proportion of normal-but-different babies treated 'successfully' in the age-group under 3 months. However, cynicism alone should not prevent early treatment. There is a *prima facie* case physiologically, anatomically and socially for the earliest possible intervention in all but the very preterm babies.

The treatment dilemma

There are children with CP for whom treatment is straightforward, simple and finite, but those with bilateral disorders now present more often with a complex developmental disability set within a troubled family and for them the treatment situation is seldom clear-cut. All too frequently a precise prognosis can only be guessed, and yet the treatment (certainly after the first year of life) must increasingly relate to the child's ultimate potential. Any treatment regime will curtail the child's freedom to some extent and so act as a separation from the normal world; yet without such help the most advantageous function as an adult may not be possible (see Chapter 12). Finding the balance is difficult.

Some families are always wanting to do more; others find even the most limited attendance or treatment too onerous. Some babies/children cooperate and enjoy treatment, others are practically unapproachable; some are at home all day, others at a day nursery or school. Each of these factors affects the possibilities of treatment. So, from the outset the treatment has to suit the child rather than the disorder.

CP poses problems unlike those encountered in many equally disabling disorders. One needs to see very many children with CP and watch them grow into adults before it is possible to appreciate the natural history of the disorder and its response to treatment. Its almost infinite variety (and the lack of a common language to describe this variety accurately) makes learning about it very difficult indeed. Personal experience is the only effective teacher but the incidence of CP is too small for experience to be easy to come by and as a result many children are treated by those with insufficient understanding of the problems. It seems to be essential that this group of disorders be supervised by those who see the children with disability from a large population, probably not less than a million overall; only then can they build up experience of managing the wide variety of problems presenting at all ages.

Few children have the possibility of the 'best' treatment for all aspects of their disorder. This is partly because no one clinic will have the expertise in all fields, but also because there is often so much that *could* be done that treatment would be disproportionate and dominate the lives of the child, parents and siblings. Unless a child is removed from the family, or the whole family is diverted to the child's advancement, treatment must become a compromise.

Finding the optimal compromise implies that the therapist has to assess (use experience to guess) the prognosis with and without treatment for each aspect of the disorder, and to decide whether that aspect of treatment is likely to be a significant benefit and, if so, whether the time needed (by the child and their family) for treatment and travel makes the outcome of *overall* benefit. For time is not on the side of the child: childhood is limited by growth and cannot be extended arbitrarily for therapeutic convenience.

Conflicting aims
It is not unusual for treatments to conflict: deformity might best be minimized by preventing certain postures or movements, but these may be disadvantageous for that one aim only and be an important part of the child's functional life. Encouraging a child to function freely and achieve is important, but is it more or less important than preventing the deformity such a function produces? Preventing a deformity might be achieved by orthotic restriction of movement, but is that more or less important to the child than self-perception or the opinion of their peers? The first dilemma of treatment is *whether* and *what* to treat; rather than *how* to do so.

'Normal' movement
Another problem is deciding the importance of the look of a movement or posture (cosmesis).

Those with CP can never move totally 'normally', but the balance between the look of a
~~~~~~ ~~~ ~~~ functional efficiency is important and the priority can vary
vever, it is important not to idealize 'normal' move-
nent goal. What we regard as 'normal' is not special
um way of functioning in this environment (air and
gths, masses, joint ranges, muscle dispositions, etc.)
. Change any one of these and the optimum way of
oon, astronauts' movements were not earth-normal,
a water, we wade: normal walking is what a person
he earth's surface. In water (and buoyancy) the efficient
ct of this difference is relevant to some children with
an extend at the knee by a pendular 'swing through',
rained by spastic hamstrings cannot, so some children
t to walk. If a hip or knee is arthrodesed, locomotion
be so. Why then is it assumed that for someone with
t should be the treatment goal? Yet many implicitly
atment results by their approximation to normal, rather
s. Conductive Education understands this and so aims
efficient way of moving (Hari and Tillemans 1984).

e of normal function, not its cause.

ed as hyper- or hypotonia, indicating that tone is a
an that the child would benefit from it being reduced
is, brought 'nearer to normal'. Obviously, tone has a
n upon that masks its other, more important, qualitative
to allow or produce 'normal' movement and posture.
ot affect this ability and may have serious negative
ral stability. An analogy might help here. If a musical
e, playing it quieter may make it less jarring on the ear,
ever quietly it is played it will never become the correct

this neuromuscular property that is almost indescribable.

iew
ed there is a danger that once treatment has started, it
it to be stopped. This is particularly true for children
ig. Their functional needs and the demands put upon
vince oneself that if function has improved then the
e; and if function is reduced, then further treatment is
ig, so are their needs. A treatment regime that was ideal
ision today. Improving emerging gait may have been a

reasonable aim, but now that the child is running about, treatment to this end may serve only to impede their social development.

Thus, treatment needs to be justified before it is started, and have precise aims and a review date; and all this should be clearly understood by the parents.

The decision not to treat is a positive one and needs careful discussion with the parents. It must be seen to be a reasonable response to their child's needs and not as indifference or neglect, and, of course, requires clearly stated periodic review.

Conluding remarks

The wide variations in types and severity of CP and the children's circumstances make any book on this subject difficult. Although this is not a book about 'how to treat' this or that type of disorder, I considered that some special mention had to be made of hemiplegia. Of course infantile hemiplegia is one of the cerebral palsies, but it is so unlike the vast majority of bilateral CP disorders in its social, emotional and functional effects on the child and future adult life as to make its management entirely different, meriting a physical treatment book of its own. I have endeavoured to explain this elsewhere (Scrutton 2000), and for the present I refer the reader to that chapter.

The authors in this book represent some of the most experienced clinicians anywhere. The editors appreciate that each chapter can only touch upon the topic in the space available, but as one reads each contribution the knowledge, experience and above all understanding of these children's problems shine through.

REFERENCES

Collis, E. (1947) *A Way of Life for the Handicapped Child*. London: Faber & Faber.
Hari, M., Tillemans, T. (1984) 'Conductive Education.' *In:* Scrutton, D. (Ed.) *Management of the Motor Disorders of Children with Cerebral Palsy. Clinics in Developmental Medicine No. 90*. London: Spastics International Medical Publications, pp. 19–35.
Scrutton, D. (2000) 'Physical assessment and aims of treatment.' *In:* Neville, B., Goodman, R. (Eds.) *Congenital Hemiplegia. Clinics in Developmental Medicine No. 150*. London: Mac Keith Press, pp. 65–80.
Slominski, A.H. (1984) 'Winthrop Phelps and the Children's Rehabilitation Institute.' *In:* Scrutton, D. (Ed.) *Management of the Motor Disorders of Children with Cerebral Palsy. Clinics in Developmental Medicine No. 90*. London: Spastics International Medical Publications, pp. 59–74.

2
THE SPECTRUM OF DISORDERS KNOWN AS CEREBRAL PALSY

Martin Bax and J. Keith Brown

The term cerebral palsy (CP) was first made popular, or begun to be used widely, in the 19th century by writers such as William Little, a surgeon (1862), Sigmund Freud (1897) and the physician William Osler (1889). It is probably Osler's book *The Cerebral Palsies of Childhood* that led to the widespread use of this term to describe children with 'palsies' that were cerebral in origin, as opposed to the other types of palsy, which can be divided into three groups: (1) orthopaedic palsies such as congenital dislocation of the hips, juvenile rheumatoid arthritis, amputations and land mine injuries; (2) muscular palsies, *e.g.* the muscular dystrophies, the myopathies and inflammatory muscular diseases; and (3) spinal palsies, *e.g.* spina bifida, spinal muscular atrophies, poliomyelitis and spinal trauma.

There have been numerous attempts at defining the cerebral palsies. One definition that has been used much in research and has stood the test of time is that reported by Bax (1964) following an international study group in Edinburgh. CP is defined as "a disorder of movement and posture due to a defect or lesion of the immature brain." It was noted that for practical purposes it is usual to exclude from CP those disorders of posture and movement that, although cerebral in origin, are: (1) of short duration; (2) due to progressive disease; or (3) due solely to, or associated with, cognitive impairment.

Certain centres restrict the term cerebral palsy to the motor (disability) that occurs from brain damage occurring before the age of 3 or 4 years. The only reason for having a condition called cerebral palsy (which is not deemed necessary by adult neurologists or rehabilitation consultants) is that the condition occurs in an organism with a still developing and growing brain so the clinical picture changes with that brain growth and this continues until the late teens. There seems to be no good reason to say that a head injury at age 3 causes CP and exactly the same injury at age 4 does not, particularly when the management is the same.

A more recent definition, agreed at an international meeting held in Brioni, Yugoslavia in 1990 (see Mutch *et al.* 1992), adds only minor qualifications: CP is "an umbrella term covering a group of non-progressive, but often changing, motor impairment syndromes secondary to lesions or anomalies of the brain arising in the early stages of its development." This emphasizes (as is implied in the earlier definition) that CP is not a disease entity. Damage to the immature brain can result from a wide variety of causes including road traffic accidents, disturbances during the birth process and perinatal stroke. Hence it is essentially a clinical definition and the groups of children are defined clinically. There is an association with the pathology but it is by no means a direct correlation, and it is dangerous to conclude that CP of a particular type is uniquely related to one particular brain pathology (Brown and Lin 1998). The essential feature is that the pathology is non-progressive. Continued brain development means the clinical picture is dynamic and may appear to progress over time, so differentiation from progressive pathology may not always be easy. Particularly in the earlier years of life the symptoms may be mimicked by metabolic diseases such as glutaric aciduria, the mitochondropathies or Lesch–Nyhan syndrome.

Brain development is most rapid in terms of physical size before 4 years but is still very incomplete with regard to learning and motor skills. About 10% of CP cases are due to postnatal brain damage.

Another feature of these definitions is that they emphasize the motor disorder, but not surprisingly, as CP is caused by 'damage' to or a defect in the immature brain, other functions are frequently involved; these are discussed later in the chapter. Indeed, virtually any function of the central nervous system may be disrupted with CP, including not only those with an associated motor element, such as speech, eating/drinking, manipulation and eye movements (Brown and Walsh 1999), but also sensory and (most importantly) learning and cognitive functions. Behavioural factors may be involved so the child can have attention deficit hyperactivity disorder, depression or an autistic spectrum disorder. Although these functions may also have an environmental background, their more frequent occurrence in the CP population compared to the normal population indicates their biological basis. So, although the diagnosis of CP is defined solely in terms of motor function, any child who has CP requires and demands the most full and careful physical and clinical examination to detect all these functional limitations.

While most would agree that progressive pathology such as tumours and degenerative brain disease should be excluded from the definition, as any treatment is obscured by the progressive nature of the causative disease, there are problems when the cause of the motor disability is known. Is a child whose brain tumour has been treated successfully surgically but who retains some residual motor disorder a 'case' of CP? What about Angelman syndrome, hydrocephalus or Dandy–Walker syndrome? Do children with these disorders have ataxic CP? Most diagnosticians would probably exclude Angelman syndrome but include hydrocephalus within the cerebral palsies.

Although some children with hemiplegia walk at similar ages as the normal population, others are slow; children with bilateral CP who walk will invariably do so late, and CP is usually characterized by delayed as well as abnormal motor activity. So how important is delayed motor development in the diagnosis? If a child has a moderate or severe learning difficulty, s/he may well not be walking at 3 years but have no signs of spasticity or paresis. All normal children when they start to walk have a broad base with flat feet, hold their arms raised ('high guard'), and have an abducted and slightly stomping gait, *i.e.* the gait of a child with ataxic CP. If this stage is delayed or prolonged does the child have ataxic CP? Again, most people would probably rule that out because the child has the possibility to develop a normal walking pattern.

The neuropathological findings are discussed later but one should try to understand the causes behind the neuropathological changes. Stanley *et al.* (2000) stress the need to think of causal pathways rather than a single disease entity, so that they describe an event such

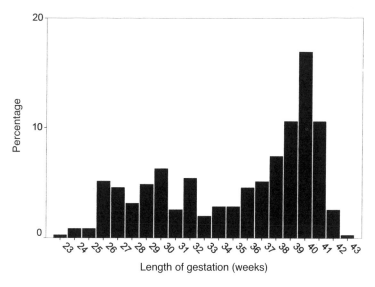

Fig. 2.1. Length of gestation of CP cases in the European Cerebral Palsy Study (n = 349) (unpublished data).

as preterm birth not as the cause of CP, but as one of the factors that has led to CP. The causal pathways may include genetic factors—for example, there are certain familial paraplegias, but possibly more importantly there may be a genetic tendency for a brain to be vulnerable. Other factors may be important here, such as the cytokines produced in inflammatory responses.

Clearly there is a wide range of commonly associated factors, of which the most important is low birthweight or being small for gestational age. Years ago any baby born before 36 weeks was a vulnerable baby but most now have good outcomes. Careful neonatal care probably prevents some 32–36 week babies from having CP who only 10–15 years ago would have developed it; and 24–28 week babies, who rarely survived 20 years ago, are now clearly seen as potential survivors deserving of intensive neonatal care. However, when these 24–28 week survivors turn up at clinics they are often the most severely affected, with 'total body' CP and profound learning difficulties. The notion that the survivors of these very early babies have dramatically increased the number of severe children with CP is problematic. Although babies born at 24–30 weeks show a much higher rate of mortality and morbidity, the numbers involved are so small that the overall effect on the rates of CP is not very significant (Fig. 2.1).

Classification of cerebral palsy

There is a long historical background to this process but essentially CP is subclassified by the nature of the motor disorder and its distribution. The distribution can be monoplegia, hemiplegia, diplegia (legs worse than arms), triplegia, and tetra- or quadriplegia (all four limbs equally affected). In practice, mono- and triplegia are rarely used. This classification

11

TABLE 2.1
Comparison of the percentages of the main topographical cerebral palsy
subtypes from two large surveys*

	Mutch and Ronald (1992) (N = 502)	European study** (N = 381)
Spastic		
Monoplegia	2	—
Hemiplegia	21	27
Diplegia	22	36
Tetra/quadriplegia	33	21
Ataxic		
Truncal	6	4
Dyskinetic/dystonic	3	12
Mixed/unclassified	13	—

*The pattern will vary with the population sampled and with regional variations in aetiological factors. A major problem is inclusion of motor disability in known diseases, as it is highly unlikely that there were no mixed cases, or only 4% of children with ataxia, in these large populations. There is a tendency to make the clkinical findings fit the classifications for epidemiological purposes. This can confuse the therapist interested in functional developmental prognosis and mechanisms of deformity. Mixed pictures such as ataxic diplegia, ataxic hemiplegia and dystonic hemiplegia, or classifying an asymmetric double hemiplegia as a simple hemiplegia, or four-limb involvement as a diplegia of tetraplegic distribution will make the prognosis for walking, bulbar involvement, mental retardation, scoliosis, hip dislocation or epilepsy, very different from the risk in a simple case.
**European Cerebral Palsy Study (unpublished data, 2003).

by distribution applies mainly to the spastic types because in general the other motor disorders have total body involvement.

The nature of spasticity is discussed elsewhere in this book but essentially the child has stiff limbs that resist movement (hypertonia), increased reflexes and 'static' postures, whereas the dystonic and athetoid groups have variable tone and unwanted movements with dynamic posturing. Classically, the postures of CP are well described (see below). Many children have a mixed pattern, *e.g.* a dystonic pattern with 'diplegia'. Table 2.1 sets out the common patterns of CP seen in Edinburgh in 1992 and in a European study of children born between 1996 and 1998 (not yet published).

Diplegia

The child described as having classical diplegic CP has slightly flexed and internally rotated hips, semi-flexed knees, extended plantar-flexed ankles, and, depending on the extent of involvement and effectiveness of management, some fixed contractures potentially at all three joints (hip, knee and ankle). There is also some associated posturing in the upper limbs with internally rotated shoulders, flexed elbows, wrists and fingers, and adducted/opposed thumbs. This pattern is often not seen until after 2 years of age and may not be completely apparent until 3 or 4 years. Early on, most commonly before the age of 1 year, there will be a dystonic phase when the child will have accompanying hypertonia and the diagnosis of CP may be quite difficult. As the child gets older, usually toward the end of the first year and during the second year, spasticity becomes more prominent. It is discouraging for the therapist to think that their treatment has failed to prevent the spastic pattern, when in fact what is happening is simply the natural history of the disease.

Hemiplegia

In hemiplegia the arm appears to be much more involved than the leg, although this is partly because the less affected proximal part of the body makes walking look relatively 'normal'. The lack of fine movement of the hand is very apparent, but fine movement of the toes is equally impaired. The characteristic postures are similar to those of diplegia but affect only half the body. Bony undergrowth of the affected limb, when present, occurs in the first two years of life (and beyond) and if not suitably managed may play a part in the development of a contracture of the tendo Achilles. What is so apparent in a unilateral disorder points to the fact that many diplegic children will have some bony undergrowth in both limbs. Virtually all children with hemiplegia walk, although their onset of walking may be delayed. Non-walking is correlated with profoundly delayed general development or epilepsy and therefore often indicates bilateral brain pathology even though the motor disability is more unilateral.

Quadriplegia

Most children with tetra- or quadriplegic distribution have very severe CP, frequently associated with seizures and severe cognitive impairment. Spasticity dominates in all four limbs. The children develop no (or very minimal) functional movement and they are at great risk of developing contractures and deformities. Unless their care throughout life is good, they are likely to develop both scoliotic and kyphotic problems in adult life.

For some infants and young children who lack postural control and show little or no ability to move, it is difficult to distinguish whether the cause is a profound motor disorder, a profound learning difficulty or a combination of both, as the motor signs of CP too are 'delayed' or overshadowed by secondary postitional disorder from immobility (Fulford and Brown 1976, Brown 1985).

Dystonic/dyskinetic CP

The term dystonic is now generally preferred to those of extrapyramidal or athetoid CP. Dystonic CP has few signs in the early months of life except possibly some variations in muscle tone, but abnormal postures and movements begin to occur in the second half of the first year. There are unwanted movements around the mouth and of the arms and legs, and these become particularly prominent when attempting fine or gross motor movements. There are very varied patterns of the abnormal movements but swallowing difficulties are common. Many of the children make odd grimacing movements of the face, which are often associated with attempted movements in other parts of the body.

Early on in the first year of life it may be difficult to distinguish between the child who is later going to be dystonic and the child with cerebral diplegia because both have a dystonic

13

phase. In the dyskinetic child the varying tone persists, and tendon reflexes tend to be normal and may be increased in the lower limbs. The child has abnormal postures with increased tone depending upon position in space, relation of head to body, contact with a surface (lying position) or stimulation of the perioral region or perineum (changing nappies). Intentional activity itself is clumsy and uncoordinated, and the unwanted movements may make effective voluntary activity impossible. In this form of CP bulbar problems are most common, swallowing difficulties are frequent and may affect nutrition, and drooling may be a major problem (although it is quite common across all groups of children with CP). Speech is always impaired with a dysarthria as a result of involvement of the muscles and may affect nutrition.

Ataxia

Table 2.1 shows that this is a much less common disorder. The child does not have unwanted movements but volitional movements are affected usually all over the body. In classical neurology there is an unsteady, wide-based stamping gait and often gross intentional tremor in the arms and hands. The infant with ataxic CP presents as a floppy baby with tonic paresis (*i.e.* reduced muscle tone), the opposite to spasticity. There are increased ranges of movement at all joints, hip abduction, straight leg raising, popliteal angles, dorsiflexion at the ankle, supination, etc. Reflexes are brisk and pendular. Postural development (rolling/sitting/standing) is delayed, as is walking. Physiological ataxia is prolonged, and speech is slow and of a developmental pattern rather than the dysarthria of acquired ataxias. Hand skills are disrupted in judging speed, distance and power, and as the cerebellum is involved in motor learning the child may appear dyspraxic.

Many cases are missed and so do not appear in CP studies. The CNS malformations such as Meckel–Gruber syndrome, vermis aplasias, Joubert syndrome, hydrocephalus and Dandy–Walker syndrome all cause an ataxia but are not included as CP. There are also a large number of genetic syndromes (mainly also eponymous) that result in ataxia (Brown and Lin 1998).

Other motor activities

Most people when considering the child with CP and motor disorders think about the movements involving the upper and lower limbs, but other motor activities are also involved. Amiel-Tison and Gosselin (2001), for example, have stressed the difficulties with trunk movements seen by children with CP. Beyond that, the two principal areas affected are those involved with the production of speech and those involved with eating and drinking. Lack of coordination of the suck/swallow and respiratory activities can mean that the child has extreme difficulty with and dislike of the feeding process. The failure to integrate swallow and breathing may mean that aspiration takes place and the child develops respiratory disease. The brain coordinates swallowing and oesophageal peristalsis, and there is a very high incidence of gastro-oesophageal reflux especially in those children with total body involvement. These problems can be so grave that it is necessary to use an alternative way of providing nutrition for the child, and the use of gastrostomy in CP has become increasingly common over the last 10 years. There are debates about its effectiveness but there is no doubting that failure to provide adequate nutrition to the baby in the early weeks and months of life may increase the extent of the neurological damage as well as causing wastage of muscles that therapy is trying to strengthen.

Speech and language

It has often been assumed that the occurrence of eating/drinking difficulties will predict the occurrence of speech problems but the association is not in fact so direct. One sees children who can speak well but who are still having great difficulty feeding, and vice versa. Dysarthric patterning of speech is most commonly seen in those children with dystonic CP. Some of these children and young people have good cognitive levels and suffer extreme frustration from being unable to communicate and this has led to the development of alternative and augmentative communication systems (Cockerill and Carroll-Few 2002).

Associated findings

As has been stressed earlier, in all these syndromic conditions additional features are often present such as epilepsy, moderate to severe learning disorders, attention deficit disorder, specific learning difficulties, perceptual problems, and autism in some cases. The patterns of these involvements tend to vary with the subclinical types so that severe epilepsies are prominent in the spastic quadripegic group of children. In all groups it is considerably above the norm, and sometimes the condition is very hard to treat. Feeding difficulties are common, particularly in the young child. Visual problems are present in varying proportions in different groups, but again are commoner in all groups than in the normal population.

Given this protean picture the condition requires a comprehensive child development centre with a broad range of staffing to deal with all the child's problems. For a fuller discussion of the management of CP see Aicardi and Bax (1998).

Pathology

When first described, CP was often thought to be associated with problems during delivery, a view propounded by Little (1862), but now it is recognized that many cases occur prenatally. In addition the notion of a single event causing the CP has been replaced by one of multifactorial causes with an end result of hypoxic damage to the nerve cells. Figure 2.2 shows the MRI findings in the multicentre European Cerebral Palsy Study currently being conducted by Martin Bax, Clare Tydeman and coworkers (unpublished data). It will be seen that the predominant pathology is periventricular leukomalacia (PVL), with cortical–subcortical damage and basal ganglia damage making up approximately a third of the cases. It is usually stated that PVL, classically associated with diplegia, is a condition resulting from preterm birth. Although that may generally be so, cases of PVL also arise among term children, with the possibility that the damage occurred several weeks before birth. The cortical–subcortical picture is often associated with severe spastic quadriplegia and in addition to the motor signs there is gross learning difficulty and high rates of epilepsy. In the dystonic group the area of damage is the basal ganglia and the condition is usually associated with quite moderate learning disorders and lower rates of epilepsy, but with very significant problems with the development of speech and language.

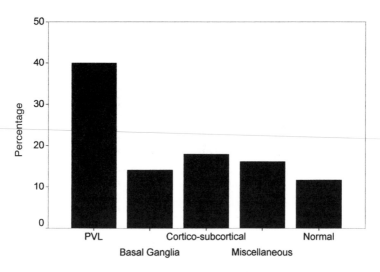

Fig. 2.2. MRI lesion pattern type among CP cases in the European Cerebral Palsy Study (N = 290) (unpublished data). PVL = periventricular leukomalacia.

The development of sophisticated neuroimaging techniques in the last two decades means that one is now able to explain to families the nature of the damage to the child's brain, and very often this may have some direct clinical relevance, although as stressed, there are not one-to-one relationships. Nevertheless, PVL is often associated with diplegia, and one can see that the white matter pathways to the spinal cord have been reduced in size, offering an explanation for the problems in the lower limbs. In the case of posterior lesions, descending pathways to the lower limbs will be affected more than those to the upper limbs. There is also a relationship between the severity of the lesion and the severity of the clinical manifestation, as illustrated in Figure 2.3. However, while these findings are useful for the clinician and informative to the parent regarding the damage that has occurred, they do not state what has caused the damage. Usually one can know only that it is an hypoxic–ischaemic insult, as the end result perhaps of a chain of events. Stanley *et al.* (2000) have stressed the importance of looking for causative pathways where one can see a pattern of events that may or may not lead to CP. The example taken from their book is of athetosis, and Figure 2.4 indicates how this process can be interrupted at various stages to prevent the development of the disability.

Our knowledge about the causes of CP is increasing; for example, we know that in many cases there is a strong association between CP and preterm birth (Forfar *et al.* 1994). Fifty per cent of children with CP are born before 36 weeks gestation, although it should be borne in mind that a very consistent figure of over 1 per 1000 children born at term have CP. We can suggest ways in which the brain can be affected during the preterm period due to, for example, the fragility of the germinal matrix at this time, causing greater likelihood of intraventricular haemorrhage, which in turn can cause any topographical type of CP (Lin *et al.* 1993). Other pathologies include infarctive periventricular leukomalacia and perinatal

16

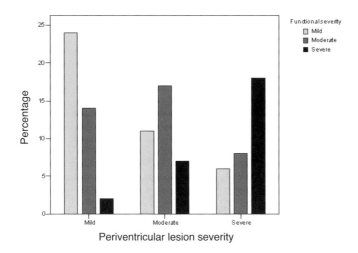

Fig. 2.3. Periventricular lesion severity *vs* functional severity among CP cases in the European Cerebral Palsy Study (N = 112) (unpublished data).

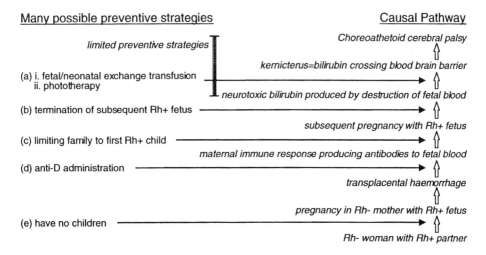

Fig. 2.4. The causal pathway to choreoathetoid cerebral palsy, and suggested preventive strategies. (Reproduced from Stanley *et al*. 2000.)

telencephalic leukoencephalopathy from presumed cytokine toxicity (Brown *et al*. 1994).

A causative factor in the hemiplegic cerebral palsies is stroke, and in Figure 2.5 we see a typical middle cerebral artery infarct pattern. Occasionally we know of a specific factor that causes such a problem, such as seen with factor V Leiden.

This very brief account of some of the factors involved in causing the pathology in CP must be extended back to include, for example, infections in pregnancy, abnormality of the

17

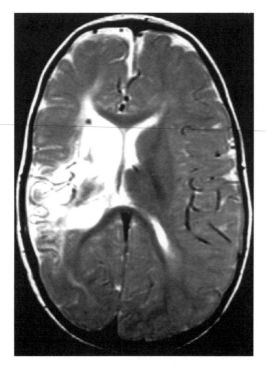

Fig. 2.5. MRI showing middle cerebral artery infarct in a 12-month-old boy with left hemiplegia.

placenta, congenital rubella, cytomegalovirus infection and maternal HIV infection, to mention just a few.

Structuring an overall plan for the management of the child with CP
The needs of a child with physical disabilities are that (1) they should be identified, then (2) a diagnosis made, (3) an assessment conducted, (4) a treatment plan and (5) a management plan proposed, (6) care and counseling given where appropriate, and (7) the situation in terms of management, diagnosis and assessment should be reviewed on a periodic basis.

Identification will often mean that the family or indeed the attendants at birth may see that something is wrong with the child where there is a clear dysmorphological feature. Equally, with many motor disorders the child may not appear abnormal at birth and symptomatology/ functional difficulties appear during the early months of life. Regular assessment, regular developmental checks and attention to parental anxieties will mean that the baby with a problem should be identified as soon as the problem can be identified. Then the child needs to be seen by somebody with enough experience to decide whether the child is within the variance of normal or has a problem. This may require some observation over time before a decision is possible. Once the child is identified as having a problem it is necessary for a diagnosis to be made; this may then have clear-cut prognostic outlines, *e.g.* the child with muscular dystrophy has a progressive disorder whereas the child with CP does not. The diagnosis will often involve investigations, but beyond that, in order to provide help for the child and family, the child's function needs to be assessed. Assessment should take regard of the fact that CP (as discussed earlier) is not a full diagnosis but rather a syndromic one. Within the syndrome there is a wide range of functional ability. In order to make the assessment, a team of therapists, educators, psychologists and health professionals will be involved as appropriate. A programme can be planned together with the family to provide the optimum health for the child, to maximize their potential.

Treatment implies a cure and in many motor disorders caused neurologically, cure is not possible. It is important to emphasize this when the child is identified and diagnosed. What one is often doing is providing 'management' where (as outlined above) the child's functional potential is maximized, but the actual neurological deficit cannot any longer be altered. That is not to say that things may not change. Errors in diagnosis occur, and ideas about treatment and management change over time. So the whole team needs, together with the family, to reassess the child at regular intervals, and that may mean going back and questioning the initial diagnosis. Then the child will need care, which is slightly different to treatment or management in that it involves seeing that the child is in an environment that allows for management programmes to be instituted. Care may involve looking at issues around housing, finances in the family, and in most countries some sort of social service provision.

A very important part of this process is what is called 'disclosure', namely the presentation to the family of the conditions that have been identified in the child. This process is difficult both for the family and for the professional advisors who need good training in how this should be carried out (*e.g.* see *Right From the Start*, Scope 1999).

The causal pathways in individual children are often difficult to establish. This is always distressing to families who very much want to know 'what went wrong'. The finding in some instances of a genetic factor is also upsetting, implying some 'defect' in the parents causing their child's problems.

The parents will want to know what the likely effects are and whether the child will or will not walk and be able to lead a 'normal' life. Having been told that CP is a disorder of movement and posture, families rightly expect help with these problems, and early on the parental demand may be for some form of motor therapy. Frequently their expectations go beyond what one considers will actually help the child. Professionals used to consider that it was their role to lay down the pattern of management for the child, but more recently the primacy of the parental role has been recognized. As recommended by McConachie *et al*. (1997), in some instances it is appropriate to meet parental demand in spite of the lack of scientific data to support it. Certain services or facilities should be available as a basic right in a caring society, rather than these having to meet a strict scientific test of effectiveness. At the same time, we live in an age of evidence-based medicine and perhaps no group of children have had so much treatment on so little evidence. Physiotherapy, occupational therapy and speech therapy although unproven probably did no harm except for endendering unrealistic parental expectations. On the other hand, major orthopaedic surgery, gastrostomy, rhizotomy, botulinum, intrathecal baclofen and basal ganglia pacing are potentially hazardous or even fatal and must be applied on an evidence base. If a child cannot walk further, faster or using less oxygen (less fatigued), then what have we achieved? Some form of objective measurement such as gait analysis, gross movement scores, or physiological measurements of tone and joint ranges should be mandatory before and after any therapy regime is introduced. Health providers have a responsibility to try to measure the effectiveness of any programmes set up for children with disabilities and to identify which treatments are ineffective. On the other hand, the availability of certain services such as early intervention is now an accepted right, even though appropriate methods of evaluation may yet be lacking.

In addition to the motor problems, while many children with CP are within a normal range of intelligence, around 50% may have learning difficulties. Behaviour problems are frequent, as are many speech and language problems, and these may be the most significant issue for the child in later childhood. Sensory problems are common, including visual acuity problems (myopia is common in very low-birthweight babies), squint, and unwanted eye movements such as nystagmus. Hearing problems used to be particularly common in children with athetoid CP. Here kernicterus specifically damages auditory pathways in the brain resulting in high-frequnecy hearing loss. Regular checks of vision and hearing are important for all children and need to be repeated at regular intervals. Assessment of the child must be ongoing, and reassessment must take place on a regular basis so that one can decide which aspects of the child's problems should be having greatest attention from the team at any particular moment in time.

The team that helps the family of a child with CP must be multidisciplinary, with representatives not only from all the therapies in health, but also educationalists and social support so that the child can be included in society (see Robards 1994).

At some stage the family will need an opportunity to discuss their feelings about the situation and to come to some understanding of the predicament that their child's biological disadvantage has given them. These issues take us far beyond the child's motor disorder but they are all part of the framework into which the management of the physical disorder has been fixed. For a more extended outline of this process, see Aicardi and Bax (1998).

CP in adolescence and adulthood

Cerebral palsy is a life-long condition, and in general life expectation once early childhood has passed is not much lower than for the normal population. Nevertheless, in adolescence and early adult life the pattern of disability may vary and certain specific problems can be identified. For example, in the dystonic group, the constant movement probably leads to the early onset of osteoarthritis. Swallowing problems often seem to increase ,and in order to maintain mobility, regular exercise with the help of a physiotherapist should continue throughout life.

All these issues are under-studied and too little is known about them. Certainly the role of the physiotherapist in managing physical disorders does not stop with adolescence but should continue as long as it is required in order to help the person with a disability.

REFERENCES

Aicardi, J., Bax, M. (1998) 'Cerebral palsy.' *In:* Aicardi, J. *Diseases of the Nervous System in Childhood, 2nd Edn.* London: Mac Keith Press, pp. 210–239.
Amiel-Tison, C., Gosselin, J. (2001) *Neurological Development From Birth to Six Years.* Baltimore: Johns Hopkins University Press.

Bax, M.C.O. (1964) 'Terminology and classification of cerebral palsy.' *Developmental Medicine and Child Neurology*, **6**, 295–307.

Brown, J.K. (1985) 'Positional deformity in children with cerebral palsy.' *Physiotherapy Practice*, **1**, 37–41.

Brown, J.K., Lin, J-P. (1998) 'Cerebral palsy.' *In:* Campbell, A.G.M., McIntosh, N. (Eds.) *Forfar and Arneil's Textbook of Paediatrics, 5th Edn.* Edinburgh: Churchill Livingstone, pp. 738–774.

Brown, J.K., Walsh, E.G. (1999) 'The neurology of the upper limb in childhood hemiplegia.' *In:* Neville, B., Goodman, R. (Eds.) *Congenital Hemiplegia. Clinics in Developmental Medicine No. 150.* London: Mac Keith Press, pp. 280–316.

Brown, J.K., Lin, J-P., Goh, W. (1994) 'Handicap and pathology of the premature brain.' *Journal of the Singapore Paediatric Society*, **36** (Suppl. 1), 49–67.

Cockerill, H., Carroll-Few, L. (Eds.) (2002) *Communicating Without Speech. Clinics in Developmental Medicine No. 156.* London: Mac Keith Press.

Forfar, J.O., Hume, R., McPhail, F.M., Maxwell, S.M., Wilkinson, E.M., Lin, J-P., Brown, J.K. (1994) 'Low birthweight: a 10-year outcome study of the continuum of reproductive casualty.' *Developmental Medicine and Child Neurology*, **36**, 1037–1048.

Freud, S. (1897) 'Die infantile Cerebrallahmung.' *In:* Nothnagel. H. (Ed.) *Specielle Pathologie und Therapie. Vol. 9, No. 3.* Vienna: Alfred Holder.

Fulford, G., Brown, J.K. (1976) 'Position as a cause of deformity in children with cerebral palsy.' *Developmental Medicine and Child Neurology*, **18**, 305–314.

Ingram, T.T.S. (1962) *Paediatric Aspects of Cerebral Palsy.* Edinburgh: E. & S. Livingstone.

Lin, J-P., Goh, W., Brown, J.K., Steers, A.J.W. (1993) 'Heterogeneity of neurological syndromes in survivors of grade 3 and 4 periventricular haemorrhage.' *Child's Nervous System*, **9**, 205–214.

Little, W.J. (1862) 'On the incidence of abnormal parturition, difficult labour, premature birth and asphyxia neonatorum on the mental and physical condition of the child, especially in relation to deformities.' *Transactions of the Obstetrical Society of London*, **3**, 293–344. (Reprinted in: *Cerebral Palsy Bulletin*, 1958, **1**, 5–34.)

McConachie, H., Smyth, D., Bax, M. (Eds.) (1997) 'Services for children with disabilities in European countries.' *Developmental Medicine and Child Neurology*, **39**, Suppl. 76.

Mutch, L., Ronald, E. (1992) *The Scottish Register of Children with a Motor Deficit of Central Origin. Report to the Chief Scientist (Scotland). K/OPR/2/2/C929.* Glasgow University, Public Health Research Unit.

Mutch, L., Alberman, E., Hagberg, B., Kodama, K., Perat, M.V. (1992) 'Cerebral palsy epidemiology: where are we now and where are we going?' *Developmental Medicine and Child Neurology*, **34**, 547–551.

Osler, W. (1889) *The Cerebral Palsies of Children.* London: H.K. Lewis. (Reprinted as *Classics in Developmental Medicine No. 1*, London: Mac Keith Press, 1987).

Robards, M.F. (1994) *Running a Team for Disabled Children and their Families. Clinics in Developmental Medicine No 130.* London: Mac Keith Press.

Scope (1999) *Right From the Start.* London: Scope.

Stanley, F.J., Blair, E., Alberman, E. (2000) *Cerebral Palsies: Epidemiology and Causal Pathways. Clinics in Developmental Medicine No. 151.* London: Mac Keith Press.

3

FAMILIES AND SERVICE PROVIDERS: FORGING EFFECTIVE CONNECTIONS, AND WHY IT MATTERS

Peter Rosenbaum

Families' needs

CHALLENGES OF RAISING A SPECIAL CHILD

Raising a child with a long-term problem of health or development can present many challenges to a family (Cadman *et al.* 1991). Beyond the usual demands of parenting, families with children with special needs often experience additional worries about the uncertainties surrounding their child's prognosis, the best ways to promote development, and how to reconcile the many and sometimes conflicting opinions they receive about the 'best' therapies. Parents often find themselves involved in ongoing contact with service 'systems' that many parents of typical children never even need to know about. For example, a child with cerebral palsy (CP) typically receives developmental therapies from a children's rehabilitation program, frequently from several different service providers. The child may need special educational considerations, necessitating negotiations with school systems. If the child and family need social service supports, for example to obtain respite services, financial help or access to recreational programs, they will need to be in contact with specialized agencies and professionals on whom they depend for help.

The primary aim of this book is to provide up-to-date information and evidence concerning the best ways to manage the functional challenges faced by children with motor impairments associated with the cerebral palsies. A parallel body of emerging thinking and research has begun to explore issues in service delivery, specifically to consider how services should be provided to families like those raising children with CP. This chapter outlines current research connecting the 'processes' of service delivery with the 'outcomes' of family well-being and satisfaction. The goal is to illustrate why all service providers need to be aware that how we work may be as important as what we actually prescribe, and may in fact enhance or detract from the best advice we have to offer.

IMPACT ON FAMILIES

Encounters with service providers may impose on families a host of pressures that can create stress, anxiety and frustration. Having to answer the same questions repeatedly over the years, or retell their child's story, or reveal personal details about family issues—all these aspects of parenting a child with special needs are known to be a source of irritation and frustration. While each new provider needs to understand the child's and family's situation, from a family's perspective the information should already be 'out there' for the new people to access without starting from the beginning once again. Parents can easily wonder whether professionals actually communicate with each other, given what they experience as the redundancy in providers' activities in history-taking, assessments of child and family, and information gathering.

Are these stresses more or less severe for parents of children with CP than for parents of children with other conditions? Almost certainly not. Are experiences like these inevitable when parents have a child requiring special attention throughout childhood? They need not be. While the focus of this book is on issues concerning children with motor disorders, there are compelling reasons to cast a wider net in considering the challenges faced by parents of children with CP. The background for doing so is explained below.

NON-CATEGORICAL APPROACH

A body of ideas (Pless and Pinkerton 1975) and research data (Stein and Jessop 1982) accumulated over the past three decades suggests strongly that a 'non-categorical' way of thinking about childhood disability (and in fact about chronic childhood illness in general) can help service providers understand the generic elements of the experience of parenting when a family is raising a child with complex special needs. Simply put, the idea is that despite the individual 'predicament' experienced as a result of each child and family's unique issues (Taylor 1982) there are a number of important common elements to parents' experiences, an understanding of which can be helpful to both families and providers. This idea may at first seem counterintuitive to health and education professionals for whom specific diagnoses and categorizations are usually the stepping-off point toward service planning and management. The non-categorical approach to issues does not negate the need to understand and manage each unique situation on its own merits. What it does do, however, is offer opportunities for service providers and planners to shape services and clinical encounters in ways that recognize that whatever the diagnosis, families' perspectives, experiences and needs are likely to be more similar than their children's conditions would suggest. The anticipation of these needs can influence both the structure and the content of clinical services for children with developmental or health conditions and their families.

The remainder of this chapter focuses on aspects of the structure and process of service provision to families of children with long-term developmental challenges, and in particular on the ways that providers can enhance the caregiving experience for families and prevent the stress and dissatisfaction often reported by parents of children with disabilities.

What do we know about coordination of care?

ELEMENTS OF SERVICES

The non-categorical approach to chronic childhood conditions speaks to commonalities of parental experience across conditions. On the other hand, to address the 'predicaments' inherent in a family's experience of childhood disability (Taylor 1982), services for children with disabilities and their families need to be individualized and built upon a problem-based approach to the evaluation and management of each family's unique issues as they perceive them. There is now an emerging set of principles and practices that can serve as a compass for service providers as they enter this territory on their journey with a new family. These principles are known as 'family-centred service' (FCS) (Dunst *et al.* 1988, Rosenbaum *et al.* 1998) and represent a constellation of values, attitudes and approaches to the organization and delivery of services to children with special health needs and their families. The ideas are grounded in research that has canvassed parental views and expectations in order to ensure that services reflect parental needs and expectations (Rosenbaum *et al.* 1992, Baine *et al.* 1995). FCS thus moves the family into the centre of the process of service planning and delivery, involving them at every step of the journey to the extent that they wish to be involved.

FCS AND THE FAMILY
It would be tempting simply to argue that there is nothing new in this notion—families have always had ultimate responsibility for the well-being of their children. Previously, however, professionals assessed and prescribed, and families were expected to follow through on (be 'compliant' with) treatment recommendations that were largely if not exclusively based on the professionals' models of disease, disability and therapy. The nature of the relationship between parents and professionals was hierarchical and therefore unbalanced. This does not mean to imply that professionals were either malevolent or controlling—only that parental and family perspectives did not traditionally play a central role in the definition of problems or the management thereof. In an FCS model of service delivery the balance has shifted fundamentally toward an equal partnership between parents—the world's experts on their child, and the constant in their child's life—and professionals, with their expertise and experience in development, disability, therapies and treatments, ways of assessing progress, etc.

FCS AND THE CHILD
Another implication of the change in emphasis inherent in an FCS model is that the child is no longer the sole focus of interest to the service provider. Traditionally, service providers have assessed and treated the child's issues, often in an effort to address the 'impairments' (WHO 2001) that interfered with function. In an important sense an FCS approach has widened the spotlight beyond (while of course still including) the child, and certainly beyond the biological dimensions of a child's problems, to acknowledge and incorporate the needs of the parents and family. This 'ecological' approach recognizes that the well-being of parents and families is important to the well-being of children with special needs, and thus includes parent and family perspectives and needs in all aspects of assessment and management of the child's condition.

FCS PRINCIPLES—WHAT DOES THIS MEAN FOR ME AS A SERVICE PROVIDER?
Three principles of FCS have been incorporated into a conceptual and practical FCS frame-work (Rosenbaum *et al.* 1998). The purpose of the model is to distill the literature into a set of ideas that relate family needs to service provider behaviours. The first principle states

that "Parents know their children best and want the best for their children." It follows from this idea that families should have the opportunity to decide on the level of their involvement in decision-making about their child's needs; and obviously, they should have the ultimate responsibility for the care of their child. For service providers a number of key behaviours that facilitate collaboration include encouraging parental decision-making at every decision point; providing information as a basis for parents to make informed decisions; and assisting parents to identify both their children's and their own needs and their personal and family strengths.

People often worry that adoption of this principle means the parents 'run the show', and that service providers are simply the parents' handmaidens. There is also a belief that parents must make all the decisions about their child and family, and that service providers have to wait until parents make up their minds. Neither of these caricatured ideas is accurate. What is true is that parents should be expected to have the opportunity—based on full knowledge of their child's situation—to be part of the process by which decisions are made concerning management of their predicaments. When parents find this process difficult, service providers should certainly help and support them in reaching decisions the family will find acceptable. The difference between current thinking and traditional approaches to care provision lies in the balance of responsibility between family and providers, and in the role that each plays in this shared process.

The second principle of FCS may sound like a truism, stating that "Families are different and unique." Service providers often see only the common elements among families (for example, how often do we speak of a 'typical' parent or child, or refer to a child's mother as "Mum" rather than as "Mrs Jones"?). We may not as easily recognize and address the individuality of each child and family. Service providers who believe in this principle respect and support parents' views and goals, and accept the diversity of each family's particular characteristics and situation. They listen attentively to the family's issues, communicate clearly at an individualized level, and above all believe and trust parents, even when a family's culture or goals differ from those of the service providers.

Thirdly it is stated that "Optimal child development occurs within a supportive family and community context: the child is affected by the stress and coping of other family members." It will be apparent that this FCS principle—in fact the whole model—is 'ecological' in recognizing and valuing the well-being of parents and families as well as the child. Thus the needs of all family members are important, and all deserve support (whether directly by the child-oriented services or through recognition of needs and referral to other services). Service providers thus should consider the psychosocial needs of all the family members (often including grandparents, as discussed below). They should build on the family's strengths, involve members of the family as the parents wish, encourage the use of community supports as well as professional services, and respect the coping styles, values and cultures of each family. This in no way implies that every member of the family should be 'treated' as part of a child's developmental intervention. It does however suggest that awareness of a family's issues, and referral to appropriate resources for support and help, can and should be part of the purview of the service providers who work with a child and family.

ROLE OF GRANDPARENTS

In this respect a particular opportunity, and one too seldom used, is to inquire about the roles and perspectives of the child's grandparents. In many families the older generation represents a source of wisdom and support, as well as a resource of time and money that can make a huge difference to the child and parents. The grandparents will often have ideas, and worries, about their grandchild's disability that are important to know about and address. They are, as well, the 'parents' of adult 'children' (the people we relate to as the child's parents), and may need support in their extended parent role as the parents of our 'patient's' parents, about whom they are worried! I am recommending that with parental agreement (and of course only then) service providers should consider involving the senior generation of the family when informing, counseling, demonstrating treatment regimens, and reviewing progress. While there is a very sparse literature on the topic of grandparental involvement in childhood disability, this author's anecdotal experience with extended families has been universally rewarding.

WHAT IS THE EVIDENCE THAT ANY OF THIS REALLY MATTERS?

In the past two decades 'health services research' has begun to address systematically the processes and content of the delivery of services. For people whose problems require them to be in contact with health, educational and other 'systems' on a long-term basis, a number of elements appear to be important. As Breslau and Mortimer (1981) showed, continuity of care—seeing the same providers over time—ranks as a particularly important issue for parents of children with chronic conditions of health or development. Perhaps unsurprisingly this element is much less important to people receiving episodic health services (Breslau 1982). Rosenbaum and colleagues reported on the elements of service delivery rated and ranked according to perceived value by parents of children with disabilities (Rosenbaum *et al.* 1992). These elements were ranked very similarly by service providers (Rosenbaum *et al.* 1992) and also by parents of children with cystic fibrosis or diabetes (Baine *et al.* 1995), supporting the 'non-categorical' perspectives discussed earlier.

One might well ask, however, whether these findings are simply evidence that providers ought to respect people and treat them well. Does any of this actually matter to families, and if so, what is the evidence?

No single study has been done to assess the direct relationship between FCS and parent or child outcomes. Such a study would be difficult because FCS is as much a philosophy and a set of attitudes as it is a prescribed mode of behaviour. Nonetheless, there is evidence relating various aspects of FCS to a variety of child and family outcomes (summarized by Rosenbaum *et al.* 1998). From the adult literature one learns that three elements of service delivery—respect, information, and continuity of care—appear to be important correlates of three outcomes—stress, satisfaction, and adherence to treatment regimens (King G. *et al.* 1996). Thus there are certainly consistent suggestions from research across the health service field that what providers do, and how they do it, does make a measurable difference to the people who experience services.

In child health a body of research begun at the *CanChild* Centre for Childhood Disability Research at McMaster University (King S. *et al.* 1996, King *et al.* 1999), and replicated elsewhere [Larsson (2000) in Sweden; McConachie and Logan (2003) in the UK; Adams (personal communication, 1991) in the USA; Donaldsdottir (personal communication, 1993) in Denmark] has begun to identify and quantify the links between 'processes' of service delivery—what providers do, and how well they do it—and 'outcomes', including parental satisfaction, stress and mental well-being. The findings are based on data acquired with the Measure of Processes of Care (MPOC) (King et al. 1995, King S. et al. 1996), a measure of family-centred services that has been shown to be reliable and valid. MPOC's five scales reflect parents' perceptions of the extent to which they have experienced partnership and enabling, provision of general information (about disability issues), provision of specific information about their child, continuity and coordination in service delivery, and respectful and supportive services. As a non-categorical measure of family-centred service MPOC has been used to measure the experiences of parents of children with a variety of neuro-developmental disabilities (King S. et al. 1996, Larsson 2000, McConachie and Logan 2003), acquired head injury (Swaine et al. 1999), and cleft lip and palate (King et al. 1997).

Research using MPOC has made it possible to identify and quantify the strength of several of the connections between providers' actions and parents' experience and valuation of those services. We have observed consistently that higher MPOC scale scores are correlated with higher reported satisfaction with services, and also with lower stress levels and better parent mental health (King S. et al. 1996, King et al. 1999). Furthermore satisfaction with services and perceptions of stress regarding those services are inversely related (King et al. 1999). Thus, to the extent that parent satisfaction is an important outcome of service programs, being family centred is clearly one of the means to that end.

What this research has shown consistently is that variations in the structure and organization of services can be recognized by parents, and valued differently from one another. For example, in one study it was shown clearly that the developmental and medical services for families of children with maxillofacial anomalies, provided in a well-coordinated early intervention program, were rated more highly by parents than services received in community-based developmental rehabilitation programs. These latter services were in turn rated more highly than services received from a variety of community agencies without apparent coordination (King et al. 1997). A recent survey of family-centred services in Ontario explored the relationship between the family-centred 'culture' of a programme and parental perceptions of the services (Law et al. 2003). Results indicated that the principal determinants of parent satisfaction with service were the family-centred culture at the organization and parent perceptions of family-centred service. Parent perceptions of family-centred service were determined by the number of places where services were received and indirectly by the number of health and development problems experienced by their child.

In the same province a survey of family-centred services (King et al. 2000) found that the more problems a child experiences (as reported by parents) the more services they are likely to receive. This in turn is strongly correlated ($r = 0.79$) with the number of sources of service used by children and families. Thus complexity of disability is associated with a great risk of fragmentation in service delivery, which is then associated with lower ratings of family-centredness of those services. Because satisfaction, parental stress and mental health, and adherence to therapies are related to perceptions of the experiences of services, there are compelling reasons to address both what is provided, and how this is done, when families receive services for their child with long-term disabilities.

Structure and content of service delivery

What does this body of research mean for people who organize and provide services to families of children with long-term developmental disabilities? Robards (1994) has outlined many practical perspectives concerning the structure, organization and management of a district disability service. While his frame of reference is based on the resources available in the UK, the systems he discusses are clearly exportable to many regions of the world.

However, what has emerged since Robards published his perspectives a decade ago are the concepts outlined in this chapter. It seems clear that, to the greatest extent possible, efforts should be made to provide coordinated services for families of children with the most complex problems, since it is exactly these families who are at risk of stress, burn-out and dissatisfaction with the services on which they depend for their child's develop-ment. These ideas present a major challenge to service providers who make decisions about what to do and how to do it for individual children and their families. In a more complex way these ideas challenge managers of services and the policy makers whose policies determine resource allocation and often resource configuration, to think in new and imaginative ways.

In discussions of the implications of providing family-centred services, it is often said that these idealistic notions are impractical in today's world. However, this assertion remains to be tested in head-to-head comparisons of various approaches to service delivery. We would argue that the best available evidence supports the need for, and value of, comprehensive community-based programs that involve parents from the start; that provide the elements of service that have been repeatedly identified as being valued by families; and that provide services in an ecologically sensitive way to recognize family well-being as a goal of the services. To accomplish these goals will require imagination, courage in the face of conservatism about service delivery and a shift beyond traditional medical thinking.

If these concepts are accepted as desirable goals, what must change in the organization of services? The first challenge will be for people to accept the principles of family-centred service as a guiding philosophy by which services are organized and practised. Evidence from colleagues in Texas (Adams, personal communication 1991) shows that it is possible both to implement a program of FCS teaching and training, and to detect significant im-provements in parents' perceptions of services following such a program. It is also possible to assess the perceptions of service providers with the Measure of Processes of Care—Service Provider version (MPOC-SP) (Woodside *et al.* 2001), a valid and reliable service provider self-assessment measure mirrored on MPOC. Thus at least some of the tools are available for the implementation and evaluation of programs to teach FCS and assess its impact on parents and service providers.

Next it will be important to question whether developmental interventions should be directed primarily at 'fixing' impairments in children with disabilities, or at promoting 'activity' and 'participation' (WHO 2001) for those children (and their families) in develop-mentally appropriate ways. This is a contentious issue, and one that often provokes much

28

discussion among developmental professionals. The scope of the controversy is beyond the purview of this chapter, but it is important to outline the issues briefly because they involve FCS principles, practices and even perhaps resource allocation to a considerable extent.

The basic issue concerns the extent to which therapies and services are targeted at the 'impairments' experienced by children with CP (or any other condition) and to what extent efforts should be directed at promoting functional adaptation. An emerging aspect of family-centred service concerns the impact of involving families (and in fact children as well) in the identification and delineation of 'functional' goals of therapy. Ketelaar *et al.* (2001) have shown that when children with CP and their families participate in defining their own functional goals they reach those goals more efficiently, and with better results, than when the goals and therapy programs are set by service providers and are based on impairment-focused aspects of disability. As yet unpublished studies from Scandinavia also suggest that involving natural 'networks' (family and community members in the child's immediate circle) in a child's therapy can be associated with important functional gains. In addition, pilot work on family-centred functional therapy (Law *et al.* 1998) and graduate studies at *CanChild* (Lammi 2002) have shown that parents are both capable of identifying 'transitional' aspects of their children's emerging abilities, and comfortable to participate in functionally oriented therapy activities.

One wonders in fact whether the advantages of an infant development program (Learningames) over conventional neurodevelopmentally based physiotherapy (NDT) for children with diplegic CP, described by Palmer *et al.* (1988), were based on the 'developmental' emphasis of the program as distinct from the impairment-based focus of the NDT. It is this author's speculation that at least part of the explanation for the success of the Learningames program compared with conventional NDT had to do with 'allowing' and encouraging children with diplegic CP to be active and as functional as possible, even if that meant walking on their toes or with poor quality gait. One might also speculate that when parents were able to see their 'disabled' child becoming functional and engaging in developmentally appropriate activities, their perception of their child changed, leading to a new awareness of their child's capacity rather than limitation. If this is an accurate interpretation of the Palmer study then an emphasis by service providers on functional achievement and the pursuit of developmentally appropriate activities becomes another way by which services can be tailored to meet families' needs.

These latter concepts raise the possibility that being family centred might mean more than simply providing services in ways that are acceptable to families in terms of the behaviours and attitudes of service providers. FCS approaches may in fact herald a new way of looking at what is important to children and families, and of involving them directly in the delineation of their goals for intervention. This approach may in turn require that we explore innovative ways, and places, for the delivery of developmental services—approaches that are ecologically sensitive and family friendly. While this suggestion in no way minimizes the role for impairment-based interventions such as the use of botulinum toxin for treating spasticity, it does speak to the need for a broader conceptualization of what we are trying to achieve in working with children with disabilities and their families. These new ideas present exciting challenges and opportunities for all concerned with childhood disability.

The one opportunity we should be certain not to miss is the chance to give thoughtful consideration—and attentive research effort—to every innovation we explore.

REFERENCES

Baine, S., Rosenbaum, P., King, S. (1995) 'Chronic childhood illnesses: what aspects of caregiving do parents value?' *Child: Care, Health and Development*, **21**, 291–304.

Breslau N. (1982) 'Continuity re-examined: differential impact on satisfaction with medical care for disabled and normal children.' *Medical Care*, **20**, 347–360.

Breslau, N., Mortimer, E.A. (1981) 'Seeing the same doctor: determinants of satisfaction with specialty care for disabled children.' *Medical Care*, **19**, 741–57.

Cadman, D., Rosenbaum, P., Boyle, M., Offord, D. (1991) 'Children with chronic illness: family and parent demographic characteristics and psychological adjustment.' *Pediatrics*, **87**, 884–889.

Dunst, C., Trivette, C., Deal, A. (1988) *Enabling and Empowering Families*. Cambridge, MA: Brookline Books.

Ketelaar, M., Vermeer, A., Hart, H., van Petegem-van Beek, E., Helders, P.J. (2001) 'Effects of a functional therapy program on motor abilities of children with cerebral palsy.' *Physical Therapy*, **81**, 1534–1545.

King, G., King, S., Rosenbaum, P. (1996) 'Interpersonal aspects of caregiving and client outcomes: a review of the literature.' *Ambulatory Child Health*, **2**, 151–160.

King, G., Rosenbaum, P., King, S. (1997) 'Evaluating family-centred service using a measure of parents' perceptions.' *Child: Care, Health and Development*, **23**, 47–62.

King, G., King, S., Rosenbaum, P., Goffin, R. (1999) 'Family-centred caregiving and well-being of parents of children with disabilities: Linking process with outcome.' *Journal of Pediatric Psychology*, **24**, 41–52.

King, S., Rosenbaum, P., King, G. (1995) *The Measure of Processes of Care (MPOC). A Means to Assess Family-Centred Behaviours of Health Care Providers*. Hamilton: McMaster University, Neurodevelopmental Clinical Research Unit.

King, S., Rosenbaum, P., King, G. (1996) 'Parents' perceptions of care-giving: development and validation of a process measure.' *Developmental Medicine and Child Neurology*, **38**, 757–772.

King, S., Kertoy, M., King, G., Rosenbaum, P., Hurley, P., Law, M. (2000) 'Children with disabilities in Ontario: A profile of children's services. Part 2: Perceptions about family-centred service delivery for children with disabilities.' Available at www.fhs.mcmaster.ca/canchild (online report).

Lammi, B.M. (2002) 'Changing the task and environment to enhance performance of children with cerebral palsy: a single subject study.' Master's thesis, McMaster University, Hamilton, Ontario.

Larsson, M. (2000) 'Organizing habilitation services: team structures and family participation.' *Child: Care, Health and Development*, **26**, 501–514.

Law, M., Darrah, J., Rosenbaum, P., Pollock, N., King, G., Russell, D., Palisano, R., Harris, S., Walter, S., Armstrong, R., Watt, J. (1998) 'Family-centred functional therapy for children with cerebral palsy: An emerging practice model.' *Physical and Occupational Therapy in Pediatrics*, **18**, 83–102.

Law, M., Hanna, S., King, G., Hurley, P., King, S., Kertoy, M., Rosenbaum, P. (2003) 'Factors affecting family-centred service delivery for children with disabilities.' *Child: Care, Health and Development*. (In press.)

McConachie, H., Logan, S. (2003) 'Validation of the Measure of Processes of Care for use where there is no Child Development Centre.' *Child: Care, Health and Development*, **29**, 35–45.

Palmer, G.B., Shapiro, B.K., Wachtel, R.C., Allen, M.C., Hiller, J.E., Harryman, S.E., Mosher, B.S., Meinert, C.L., Capute, A.J. (1988) 'The effects of physical therapy on cerebral palsy: A controlled trial in infants with cerebral palsy.' *New England Journal of Medicine*, **318**, 803–808.

Pless, I.B., Pinkerton, P. (1975) *Chronic Childhood Disorder. Promoting Patterns of Adjustment*. London: Kimpton.

Robards, M.F. (1994) *Running a Team for Disabled Children and Their Families. Clinics in Developmental Medicine No. 130*. London: Mac Keith Press.

Rosenbaum, P., King, S.M., Cadman, D. (1992) 'Measuring processes of caregiving to physically disabled children and families. Part I: Identifying relevant components of care.' *Developmental Medicine and Child Neurology*, **34**, 103–114.

Rosenbaum, P., King, S., Law, M., King, G., Evans, J. (1998) 'Family-centred services: A conceptual framework and research review.' *Physical and Occupational Therapy in Pediatrics*, **18**, 1–20.

Stein, R.E.K., Jessop, D (1982) 'A non-categorical approach to chronic childhood illness.' *Public Health Reports*, **97**, 354–362.

Swaine, B.R., Pless, I.B., Friedman, D.S., Montes, J.L. (1999) 'Using the measure of processes of care with parents of children hospitalized for head injury.' *American Journal of Physical Medicine and Rehabilitation*, **78**, 323–329.

Taylor, D.C. (1982) 'The components of sickness: diseases, illnesses and predicaments.' *In:* Apley, J., Ounsted, C. (Eds.) *One Child*. London: Heinemann, pp. 1–13.

Woodside, J., Rosenbaum, P., King, S., King, G. (2001) 'A measure of processes of care for service providers: development and properties of a self-report measure.' *Children's Health Care*, **30**, 237–252.

WHO (2001) *International Classification of Impairment, Activity and Participation—ICIDH-2*. Geneva: World Health Organization.

4
GOAL SETTING AND THE MEASUREMENT OF CHANGE

Eva Bower

What is a goal?

One definition of a goal according to *Webster's New International Dictionary* is 'the end of a race or a journey', or to put it another way, the end-point of an objective. Other definitions are related to a variety of competitive ball games, and in these instances the number of actual goals is quantifiable. In the context of the physical management of children with cerebral palsy (CP) it is possible that a goal should be defined as a standard of activity, probably but not necessarily motor, against which an observation of the child's performance can be quantified. This is similar to Wade's (1992) definition of measurement. The goal itself therefore needs to be quantifiable but is not necessarily the end-point of the intervention. An example of such a goal could be 'stand holding on to the back of a chair with two hands for one minute', so that if a child achieved 30 seconds from a baseline measurement of 0 seconds a score of 50% would be allocated. If a child achieved 45 seconds from a baseline measurement of 0 seconds a score of 75% would be allocated and so on. The progress of such goals can be plotted on a graph (Fig. 4.1).

Goals need to be formulated in such a way that there is no doubt as to the extent to which they have been achieved when performance is reviewed (Bower and McLellan 1992). Therefore these goals need to be specific and measurable. In these terms, goals are different from aims. Aims reflect the general direction of changes in a child's performance. Aims do not define achievement with any measurable precision. An example of an aim could be 'improvement of trunk balance', which is not objectively quantifiable either at baseline or when performance is reviewed.

Herbert (1987), a psychologist, suggested that a workable goal was an accomplishment that helped the individual manage problematic situations. In this context, goals were really achieved when the children and/or their families had acquired the skills, practised them and employed them to solve or manage disabilities. These goals would have to be evaluated longitudinally over time and in a variety of environments.

For the purpose of this chapter a goal is defined as a precise, specific and measurable objective.

Why set goals?

Setting goals in the context of children with CP should be at the centre of attempts by therapists to reduce 'activity limitations' and resolve 'participation restrictions'. Setting goals and undertaking interventions is unlikely to normalize the neurological impairment, although

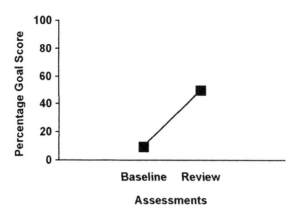

Fig. 4.1. Graph to show the progress of a goal from a baseline score of 10% to a first review score of 50%.

compensatory strategies may be adopted. The International Classification of Functioning, Disability and Health (ICIDH-2, WHO 2002) defines 'activity' as the execution of a task or action by an individual, and 'activity limitation' as difficulties an individual may have in executing activities. An example of an activity might be independent walking or upright mobility, and of activity limitation, the inability to walk or to be mobile in the upright position independently. The activity limitation might be resolved by the provision of a walking aid or a self-propelled wheelchair. 'Participation' is defined as involvement in a life situation, and 'participation restriction' as problems an individual may experience in involvement in life situations. An example of participation might be going to the supermarket to choose one's own food or being able go out of the house independently, and of participation restriction, being unable to go to the supermarket or being unable to go out of the house independently. The participation restriction might be resolved by installing a stairlift and ramps to enable the person to go down the stairs and out of the house to the supermarket to choose their own food independently.

Randomized controlled trials have to date failed to provide generalizable evidence for the effectiveness of physical therapy interventions in children with CP. As yet no single school of treatment, training or management has been proven to be more successful than any other, nor indeed has any mixture of approaches (Bower and McLellan 1994a). Treatment is usually considered to involve 'hands on' activity undertaken by the therapist. Training usually involves the child undertaking most of the activity her/himself, and management usually involves supervision by the therapist of activities undertaken by the carer and child (Bower 1999).

Many problems can complicate the undertaking of group trials to evaluate the effect of physical therapy, whether treatment, training or management, in children with CP. First, it is difficult to predict precise outcomes. What will children's future functions be? These functions are highly likely to be dependent upon the children's future environments. Will children be able to integrate socially? This is likely to be dependent upon the children's future opportunities. Can individual complications be avoided, such as the long-term insidious development of musculoskeletal deformity? This problem is still largely unresolved in the long term.

Second, rehabilitation is essentially an educational or learning process that requires active participation from each child to achieve a set of objectives or goals individual and unique to that child, unlike a pharmacological process to achieve a biological norm.

Third, it is unlikely that either the individual therapies given (what is done) or the therapists giving the therapies (who does it) are totally similar between individual participants. Each will have individual characteristics and empathies (Bower and McLellan 1994b).

In the current climate of accountability and evidence-based practice it may therefore be increasingly necessary for therapists to undertake scientifically controlled single case studies routinely in their clinical practice to demonstrate whether change has occurred over time in an individual child. This could be achieved by setting specific and measurable treatment, training or management goals for each individual child and evaluating them over time. The results might help parents, teachers, carers and even therapists to appreciate what a child can do, what a child does do, and what a child's neurological mechanisms may not yet, or ever, be ready to do. The child often knows her/his limitations perfectly well, and lack of cooperation on the part of the child often reflects this fact. Therefore the best goals are those that are realistically achievable by the child so that the child experiences success, and not failure, and parents, teachers, carers and therapists appreciate that not achieving the impossible is not failure.

If therapists wish to establish that change has, or has not, occurred as a result of intervention, additional controls need to be included. A single case study with individual goal-setting, an appropriately developed and validated outcome measure that reflects the objective of the goals set, and randomized treatment periods could be used to control for change due to maturation or spontaneous recovery and to check for the maintenance of any change observed (Bower and McLellan 1992) Figure 4.2 illustrates the design of such a procedure.

Herbert (1987) suggested that goal-setting can help children and parents in four ways: (1) by focusing attention and action, providing a vision that offers hope and an outlet for concentrated effort; (2) by mobilizing energy and helping pull children and/or parents out of the inertia of helplessness and depression; (3) by enhancing the persistence needed for working at problems; and (4) by motivating all concerned to search for strategies to accomplish them.

These suggestions are all laudable and probably help the parents more than the children. It is important not to push children too hard and not to waste time on unattainable tasks. It is unrealistic to expect children to perform at the maximum of their potential all the time, especially if it becomes a struggle for them. Most people function at the maximum of their potential only on particular occasions. Most people function at a potential with which they feel comfortable and this is equally applicable to children with CP. Goal-setting is useful because it can indicate to all concerned when there is no longer any progress and when it is therefore advisable to stop pushing the child towards that goal and just try to maintain the standard achieved, provided the child feels comfortable with that standard.

It has been shown that over short periods of two weeks (Bower *et al*. 1996), three weeks (Bower and McLellan 1992) and five weeks (Bower and McLellan 1994c) of goal-

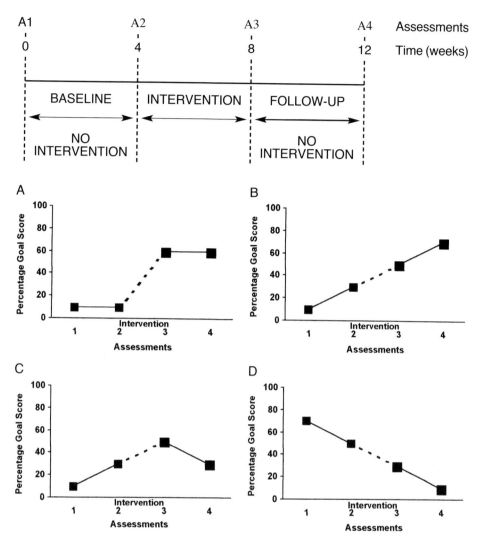

Fig. 4.2. Design to establish if change has occurred as a result of intervention. Results of assessments can be plotted on a graph and indicate (A) when improvement has occurred as a result of intervention; (B) when improvement has not occurred as a result of intervention; (C) when improvement achieved during intervention has not been maintained; or (D) when deterioration has occurred that is unchanged by the intervention.

directed therapy, improvement in gross motor function occurred. In a longer randomized controlled trial with a six-month period of goal-directed therapy (Bower *et al.* 2001) incorporating a baseline period to control for maturation and a follow-up period to control for maintenance, goal-setting procedures were not shown to have a detectable effect upon the acquisition of gross motor function or performance.

Probably the most important reason for setting goals is to make decisions about individual children. It is suggested that treatment, training or management should relate to problems experienced by the individual child and their family and that goals should reflect the objective of the therapy. Setting treatment, training or management goals traditionally provides a structure for intervention and assists with evaluation of outcome.

What is a measure?

A measure is a standard against which an observation can be quantified (Wade 1992). Examples of a standard could be a tape measure, a stop watch, a goniometer or a validated functional scale.

The difference between a goal and a measure

In the context of the physical measurement of children with CP a goal is an individual standard of activity pertinent to a particular child at a particular time, against which an observation of that child's performance can be quantified at that particular time.

In contrast, a measure is a more general standard. A measure should be appropriately developed and validated for a defined purpose with a specified population against which observations of any child or children in that population can be quantified at any time.

Why measure?

Russell and Rosenbaum (personal communication 1995) suggested that there are five main reasons for taking measurements:

1. *Individual child decision making*. What should be done with an individual child at a particular time?
2. *Effectiveness of interventions*. Is the intervention strategy effective? Is one strategy superior to another?
3. *Programme evaluation*. Are the delivery arrangements of the service satisfactory? Issues of frequency, duration, location and implementation are relevant.
4. *Quality management*. Are the recipients of the service satisfied?
5. *Professional and financial accountability*. Are time, expertise and money being used wisely?

Kirschner and Guyatt (1985) suggested that there are three main purposes for clinical measurement. In the context of physical therapy for children with CP these can be described as:

1. To ascertain if there is a motor problem and if so to describe it, that is to discriminate from the norm. One example of a discriminatory measure that is norm referenced is the Bayley Scales of Infant Development (BSID-II) Motor Scale (Bayley 1993), which assesses the developmental status of motor skills (degree of body control, large muscle coordination, fine manipulative skills of hands and fingers, dynamic movement, dynamic praxis, postural imitation and stereognosis) in children from 1 to 42 months of age to identify possible delays. It takes between 10 and 20 minutes to administer by a qualified therapist using the instruction manual.
2. To determine what the future status is likely to be in terms of motor ability, that is, to predict. There are very few validated predictive scales in the field of CP. 'Cerebral palsy'

is an umbrella term covering a very wide spectrum of disorders. Predictive scales need to be tested on a very large number of defined subjects over a long period of time which is difficult in these circumstances.

3. To assess whether change in motor activity has occurred over time, or to evaluate. One example of an evaluative measure, which is in fact also norm referenced (although for evaluative purposes a measure only needs to be criterion referenced and responsive to change), is the Paediatric Evaluation of Disability Inventory (PEDI) (Haley *et al.* 1992), which assesses adaptive function (self-care, mobility and social function) in children aged 6 months to 7 years to evaluate change over time. It takes between 45 and 60 minutes to administer by a qualified therapist using report (not observation) with an instruction manual.

Properties of measures

Different measures may have different levels of scoring, which may require different methods of statistical analysis.

Nominal scoring categorizes objects or events into groups, *e.g.* ambulant children and non-ambulant children or manual and electric wheelchairs.

Ordinal scoring is numbered in an order of value but the difference between each of the numbered values is not necessarily the same. For example, in the 88-item Gross Motor Function Measure (GMFM-88: Russell *et al.* 2002) a score of 1 = less than 10% of a task achieved whereas a score of 2 = between 10% and 99% and a score of 3 = 100% of the task achieved.

Interval scoring is numbered in an order of value but the difference between each of the numbered values is the same. For example, the difference between 1 and 2 centimetres is the same as the difference between 10 and 11 centimetres. Similarly, in the 66-item Gross Function Measure (GMFM-66: Russell *et al.* 2002), which has undergone Rasch analysis, the difference between scoring 1 and 2 or 2 and 3 is the same in terms of difficulty.

Measures should be standardized, reliable, valid and responsive.

STANDARDIZATION

Standardization of a measure should assure that all users administer and score the measure in the same way. A manual that gives clear, explicit instructions usually facilitates this process, as does training in the use of a measure.

RELIABILITY

Reliability of a measure should ensure that different users or the same user at different times produce dependable, consistently reproducible results with the same child. Training to a criterion standard and testing should facilitate this process. Inter-rater reliability concerns two people using the same measure in similar circumstances. Intra-rater reliability concerns one person using the same measure at different times. Test–retest reliability concerns the child getting the same results on two consecutive occasions. The appropriate statistics to use for testing agreement between two testers are those described by Bland and Altman (1986), called Limits of Agreement and Coefficient of Variation.

VALIDITY

Validity of a measure concerns whether a scale measures what it purports to measure. Construct validity is concerned with the purpose of the measure and whether the measure fulfils that purpose; for example, does the Pediatric Evaluation of Disability Inventory (PEDI) evaluate change over time in activities of daily living? Content validity is concerned with the items included in the measure and whether they have the potential to show change. Criterion-related validity is concerned with how the measure compares with the gold standard; for example, how does the more recently developed Peabody Development Motor Scales, 2nd Edition (PDMS-2: Folio and Fewell 2000) compare with the earlier Gross Motor Function Measure (Russell *et al*. 1993)?

RESPONSIVENESS

Responsiveness of a measure is concerned with sensitivity to change over time and is especially important in an evaluative measure.

Criteria for reviewing measures

Gowland *et al*. (1991) suggested that measures should be considered under the following headings prior to clinical use to ensure that they are suitable for the intended purpose.

• *Purpose and population*. What is the primary purpose for which the measure was designed? For which disorder, age group and cognitive ability was the measure designed?

• *Clinical utility*. Are the instructions clear and user friendly? What does the measure cost? How long does it take to administer? What is the format? What qualification or training does the examiner need?

• *Scale construction*. Are the items well selected? What is the level of measurement?

• *Standardization*. Is there a manual?

• *Reliability*. Have studies been undertaken? Were appropriate statistics used? What is the reported level of reliability?

• *Validity*. Have studies been undertaken? Is the measure responsive? Is there construct, content and criterion related validity?

How to set goals

Goal setting involves identifying and formulating standards of motor activity which are in advance of the child's current capacity or which retard deterioration (Bower and McLellan 1994a). This description, in its current form, is only relevant to motor activity. Physical therapy can target other aspects and the description can be adjusted accordingly.

The process of goal setting consists of assessing the child, setting goals, undertaking the intervention and after a set time period evaluating the goals to ascertain to what extent they have been achieved.

Assessing the child should include consideration of aspects such as their (a) likes and dislikes, (b) personality, (c) social skills, (d) daytime activities at home and at nursery/school, (e) functional abilities, (f) cognitive skills, and (g) sensory skills, in addition to all the usual motor assessments.

Goals must reflect the object of the intervention to be undertaken. For example, a boy who had recently transferred to a large local senior school with much longer distances to be covered and steeper ramps to be negotiated than in his small local junior school was experiencing particular difficulty getting himself up the ramps in his self-propelled wheelchair and was therefore frequently late for his lessons. He needed to be independent to stay at the school, which was appropriate to his cognitive abilities and enabled him to mix socially with peers living near to his home. The following options are open to him: (1) strength and endurance muscle training for his upper limbs; (2) recruit a friend to push him; (3) obtain a lighter self-propelled wheelchair; (4) obtain an electric wheelchair.

In conjunction with his physical therapist he decided to settle for options 1 and 4, and the following goals were therefore set.

SHORT-TERM GOAL
Arrive at classroom on time for daily mathematics lesson in self-propelled wheelchair using the ramp for four weeks.
Baseline = 0% always late.
Intervention: Strength and endurance muscle training for the upper limbs, supervised by the physiotherapist for 20 minutes Monday to Friday (five times weekly) at school for four weeks.
Score: 1st week – 8% per day arriving on time, whole week = 40%
2nd week – 6% per day arriving on time, whole week = 30%
3rd week – 4% per day arriving on time, whole week = 20%
4th week – 2% per day arriving on time, whole week = 10%

LONG-TERM GOAL
(a) Obtain literature describing various electric wheelchairs. Discuss.
(b) Try out these wheelchairs with boy and family at an assessment centre.
(c) Measure the boy for the most acceptable wheelchair and decide upon appropriate accessories.
(d) Order wheelchair and accessories.
(e) Accept delivery of the wheelchair for the boy and train him in its use at school.
All in 12 weeks.
Baseline = 0% no wheelchair provision.
Intervention: Proceed through stages (a) to (e) of the goal as efficiently as possible.
Score: 20% for each stage achieved under 12 weeks.

Psychologists use goal-setting to solve the problems of individual children and their families. Educationalists use goal-setting to motivate children towards a particular objective and to provide a system of monitoring towards that objective. It is suggested that in physical therapy:
1. The child needs to understand the purpose of the goal and to wish to achieve it. Therefore an understanding by the therapist of the child's motivational, cognitive and social abilities is required. Motor change may be the result of biological, intellectual, emotional or psychological change.

2. The carers need to identify the goal as a useful skill not requiring increased assistance from them. Therefore a knowledge of the home and nursery/school environments is required.
3. The therapist needs to assess that the goal can be realistically achieved. Therefore knowledge of the natural history of the disorder is required.

Occasionally the recognition of a problem and the setting of a goal provides an immediate resolution of the problem and an immediate achievement of the goal. This may occur, for example, with the provision of a piece of equipment such as a bath aid that is readily available.

When setting goals it may be helpful to consider the following points.
1. It is unlikely that physical therapy intervention can change a child from 'cannot do' to 'can do' if the neural mechanisms are not ready, in other words you are unlikely to be able to change or normalize the neurological impairment (McGraw 1943).
2. It may be possible to help the child to change from 'can do' to 'does do' if and when the child displays the wish to do so (McGraw 1943).
3. If the time window is missed during which the child wants to achieve a skill, and the necessary environment or compensatory mechanical devices have not been provided, it may be more difficult for the child to achieve that skill at a later date. Illingworth and Lister (1964) suggested that if babies were not provided with solid foods soon after they were able to chew (usually at 6–7 months) it became increasingly difficult to introduce solids later. The chronological age may vary between children with respect to these sensitive periods and is probably influenced by genetic heritage, so that a child who talks late will often have a parent who talked late and the sensitive period may also be late.
4. Children achieve skills in stages, and so goals should be formulated in simple small achievable steps allowing the child to experience success instead of failure. Cotton (1980) described a number of small steps to achieve the task of 'drinking from a cup'. The first step was 'sitting on a chair, feet flat on the floor and two hands placed on the table'. The second step was 'raising both hands to touch the ear on the relevant hand side'. The third step was 'grasping a two-handled mug placed on the table with two hands' and the fourth step was 'lifting the two-handled mug with two hands to the mouth'.
5. The secondary biomechanical constraints that result from compensatory strategies used by the child and strategies that may combat these further impairments may be valuable goals to assist in development. Whether abnormalities in muscle tone, primitive reflexes and the myotactic reflex or abnormal changes in connective tissues, muscles, bones and the rate of bone growth relative to muscle growth can be influenced by physical therapy in the long term is still controversial (Bower 1997).

Collaborative goal setting

Collaborative goal setting involves the identification of problems to be undertaken by the child, parent and nursery or school teachers and carers. This fits in well with the approach pioneered by Eirene Collis (1947) and encouraged by the Bobaths of involving parents and carers in their child's treatment and with the current concept of client-centred practice.

The likely causes of and possible solutions to these problems are then discussed between the child, the parents, the relevant teachers and carers, and the therapist. Realistic goals are

Discussion and documentation of problems with child, family, school/nursery carers and therapist

↓

Combined assessment (with people listed above) of child's:

1. likes and dislikes	2. personality	3. social skills
4. day activities (home)	5. day activities (school)	6. daily living functional abilities
7. cognition	8. hearing	9. communication
10. vision	11. fine motor	12. gross motor
13. habitual static positions and dynamic movement patterns	14. active and passive ranges of movement	

↓

Taking into account the assessment, problems documented above are jointly categorized into:

(a) those which physical therapy may help
(b) those which physical therapy may not help
(c) those which someone else may help

↓

Categorized problems (from above) are jointly ranked into priority order and documented

↓

Child, family, school/nursery carers and therapists agree on useful, realistic short-term goals and time scale in which they should be achieved — documented

↓

Physical therapist identifies their ideas on progression and long-term goals — jointly discussed and documented

↓

Realistic intervention is discussed, jointly agreed and documented

↓

Realistic frequency and duration of intervention, including who is going to carry it out, is discussed, jointly agreed and documented

↓

Measuring methods discussed, agreed and documented

↓

Child baselined on measures in presence of family/carers prior to commencement of intervention — documented

↓

Intervention commenced as agreed — progress documented

↓

Child reassessed after agreed time scale in which goals were to have been achieved – results documented

↓

Reappraisal by combined discussion

Fig. 4.3. Flow chart of procedures in the collaborative goal setting process.

```
NAME . . . . . . . . . . . . . . . . . . . . . . .         DATE . . . . . . . . . . . . . . .

PROVISIONAL DIAGNOSIS:                      CHRONOLOGICAL AGE . . . . . . . . . .

                                            DEVELOPMENTAL
                                            MOTOR AGE . . . . . . . . .


PROBLEMS (as identified by child/carers):   REASONS (as identified by therapist):




SHORT-TERM GOALS (as negotiated             LONG-TERM GOALS (as identified by
between child/carers/therapist):            therapist):




INTERVENTION (as agreed):



FREQUENCY (as agreed):



DURATION (as agreed):



MEASURES (as agreed):



BASELINE SHORT-TERM GOAL SCORES:


HAS INTERVENTION OCCURRED AS AGREED?   ☐Yes   ☐No   ☐Some doubt

REVIEW SHORT-TERM GOAL SCORES (after agreed time scale):


FURTHER ACTION (following joint discussion):
```

Fig. 4.4. Clinical physical therapy form.

42

then set together. A time scale in which the goals are to be achieved is agreed. If appropriate treatment training or management is available that is acceptable to the child, family and carers, this can be instituted and monitored by all the participants who also participate in judging the success of the intervention at goal review. This entire process should be undertaken in the child's habitual environment as pioneered in England by Eirene Collis at Queen Mary's Hospital for Sick Children, Carshalton, Surrey, and Ronnie Mac Keith at Guy's Hospital, London, and this fits in well with the current concept of community-based rehabilitation. Figure 4.3 illustrates, in flow-chart form, the procedures in the collaborative goal-setting process. Figure 4.4 is a sample form that could be used for the process.

Collaborative goal setting helps to address the immediate concerns of the child, parents and carers, in addition to enabling a gradual awareness to develop concerning what the child may or may not be likely to achieve in the longer term. It enables discussion of prognosis and intervention options. It requires a professional with sensitive interpersonal skills who understands the disorder and its likely progression (Bower 1997). An illustration of this point relates to a 6-year-old boy with CP who was able to ambulate at home and within school using an aid, whose parents expected him to learn to ride a bicycle and roller skate as a result of six months of daily goal-directed therapy. Following discussion these two goals were modified to walking up and down 10 steps independently holding one available stair rail with one hand. The ability to undertake this motor function reliably enabled this boy to go swimming each week with his school class even if a classroom assistant was not available.

Different categories of goals

In an early pilot study (Bower and McLellan 1992) goals were found to fit into three broad categories. The first category was called 'achieve a state' and was mainly concerned with relationships between children and their parents and carers. These relationships seemed to be primarily dependent upon comfort and ease in handling during daily living situations. Intervention was often by demonstration and practice of passive corrective handling and positioning of children. The techniques used were often influenced by Bobath methods, and many are well described by Finnie (1997).

An example of goal setting in this category was that of a 4-year-old girl with CP whose developmental motor age was under 6 weeks. She attended a special school. She had no demonstrable situational understanding, had epilepsy, was cortically blind, incontinent, fed by tube and tended to have respiratory problems. She cried a lot and disliked the prone position. This was thought to be due to apprehension. Her parents found that she was difficult to handle for washing and dressing as her shoulders and arms were flexed and stiff. Her therapist thought this might be helped by frequent changes of position that might accustom her to being handled and moved.

GOAL
Lie prone over a wedge with shoulders and arms extended, arm gaiters on, and fingers spread out on the floor, and tolerate for 10 minutes without crying.
Timescale: Review in three weeks.

43

Baseline = Tolerates one minute without crying = 10%.
Intervention: Position over wedge four times daily for three weeks.
Score: 10% for each minute tolerated at review.

The second category was called 'establish a daily programme' and was mainly concerned with the use of equipment and generalization of activities. These goals were often facilitated by effective equipment, demonstration and ongoing interest on the part of the therapist. Strategies such as star charts were often used to monitor compliance with regimes. An example of goal setting in this category was that of a 9-year-old boy with CP whose developmental motor age was below 15 months. He attended a special school and had cognitive, communication and visual problems. He had had bilateral adductor tenotomies and derotational osteotomies. He could ambulate wearing long leg braces with a pelvic waistband using a rollator. His learning support assistant was concerned that he rarely brought his braces to school and crawled around the classroom, using a self-propelled wheelchair in the corridors and playground. She felt that the use of his braces would enhance his dignity and avoid further hip, knee and foot deformities. His therapist agreed.

GOALS
(a) Communicate with child, parents and transport chaperone concerning current suitability of braces, problems concerning donning and doffing, toileting and carriage of braces.
(b) Bring braces to school daily.
(c) Wear braces at school all day except from 11.30 a.m. to 1.30 p.m.
(d) Stand with braces on from 9 a.m. to 10 a.m. at school.
(e) Walk with braces on from 10.00 a.m. to 11.30 a.m. and from 2 p.m. to 3 p.m. instead of using wheelchair.
Timescale: Review in four weeks.
Baseline = Lack of communication with home. Does not bring braces to school = 0%.
Intervention: Communicate with child, parents and transport chaperone. Check suitability of braces, toileting routine and problems with donning and doffing braces. Proceed through stages (b) to (e).
Score: 20% for each stage achieved at review.

The third category was called 'achieve a motor skill' and was mainly concerned with motor skill acquisition. These goals were often facilitated by repeated active movement and skill training along functional lines. Motor rehabilitation can be divided into activities that are concerned with 'whether' a child performs a motor function, those that are concerned with 'how' a child performs a motor function, and those that are concerned with both 'whether' and 'how'. 'Does the child weight bear?' is an example of 'whether' a child performs a motor function.

'Does the child flex, internally rotate and adduct at the hip when weightbearing?' is an example of 'how' a child performs a motor function. This latter aspect may be important in the delay or prevention of developmental deformity or secondary biomechanical constraints (O'Dwyer *et al*. 1989) but is more difficult to evaluate (Bower and McLellan 1994c, Bower *et al*. 2001).

An example of goal setting in this category concerned with 'whether' a child performed a motor function was that of a 3-year-old boy with CP whose developmental motor age was below 9 months. He attended a mainstream nursery school that catered for children with physical disabilities. He was cognitively intact and had no problems with vision or hearing. He did have some dysarthria and drooling problems. His right side was more affected than his left side, and his left arm was relatively unaffected. His method of mobility was commando crawling. His therapist thought that he had the potential to ambulate with a rollator if he could manage to move each leg independently.

GOAL
Stand holding on to a bar with both hands forward, lift alternate legs up on to a 4 cm thick book and down again independently.
Timescale: Review in five weeks.
Baseline = Standing holding on to a bar with both hands forwards needed help from his therapist at the pelvis and knees to lift either leg up on to a 4 cm thick book and down again = 10%.
Intervention: Repeated practice of independent leg movements in lying, sitting and standing using passive, assisted active and active movements.
Score: Lift left leg up = 20% at review
         Left leg down = 20% at review
         Lift right leg up = 25% at review
         Right leg down = 25% at review

An example of goal setting in the category concerned with 'how' a child performs relates to the same child discussed above. His therapist was concerned with the development of hip, pelvic and spinal deformity in addition to concerns over weight shift and use of his right arm.

GOAL (underlining = 'how' performed)
In high kneeling position at a table (*with legs abducted*), support himself independently with his right arm/hand and play with a toy with his left hand *while maintaining a level pelvis* for 45 seconds.
Timescale: Review in five weeks.
Baseline = In high kneeling position at a table (with legs abducted) could support himself independently with his right arm/hand and play with a toy with his left hand while maintaining a level pelvis for 5 seconds = 10%.
Intervention: Repeated practice of:
1. holding on and grasping with right hand
2. exercises to strengthen trunk and pelvic muscles
3. exercises to facilitate weight shift from right to left.

45

Score: 15% for first five extra seconds achieved at review

15% for second five seconds achieved at review

10% for each further five seconds achieved at review.

Aspects to be considered when setting goals

Goals should not only match the child's daily life but also be age appropriate. Many of the children will be delayed in motor and other abilities but their bodies will still develop, grow and reach maturity. As a result they and their families will have needs that will change over time. As suggested by Cogher *et al.* (1992):

• Young children need to be considered at home with their families. Their likely priority areas when setting goals will be family interaction, play and care routines.

• School-aged children need to be considered at school amongst their peers. Their likely priority areas when setting goals will be peer interaction, access to academic learning and functional independence.

• Adolescents and young adults need to be considered in the community and work place amongst friends, spouses and colleagues. Their likely priority areas when setting goals will be adult peer relationships, an occupation and the establishment of a role in the community.

As mentioned earlier no single treatment, training or management method has yet been scientifically proven to be generalizably superior to any other nor indeed has any mixture of approaches. It is consequently difficult to recommend any general principles for setting goals for children with CP. The following opinions, which are not supported by evidence-based trials, are, however, put forward:

• Young children, especially below the age of 2 years when pruning of unused synapses seems to take place (Greenhough *et al.* 1987) might benefit from stimulation to undertake age-appropriate activities. This applies to both normally and abnormally developing children. An example of an intervention for this age group might be to place the child on the kitchen floor near to a floor-level cupboard filled with saucepans and saucepan lids and leave the child to get to it.

• Children with milder disability, that is community and household ambulators, with or without aids, might need help to keep fit (just like many of their more normally developing peers). Problems of obesity and osteoporosis might be ameliorated. Bicycling, with an adapted bicycle if necessary, and swimming might be appropriate activities.

• Children with moderate disability, that is those who have floor mobility and usually the ability to self-propel wheelchairs indoors, might need help with problem-solving strategies, particularly for functional activities such as the use of a two handled mug for drinking, or sitting on the floor leaning against a wall in the corner of the room for support each side in order to put on shoes.

• Children with substantial disability and their families may need help with managing daily living activities such as through the provision of a hoist at home to protect the carers' backs, or frequent passive extension of soft tissues and joints to enhance joint flexibility and counteract soft-tissue stiffness.

When formulating goals it is important to ensure that: (1) they are realistic in terms of what is achievable within the limits imposed by the neurological impairment; (2) they reflect the child's wish to change; and (3) they are appropriate for the child's current environment and chronological age.

Combining goal-setting with the use of measures

Bower and McLellan (1992, 1994) and Bower *et al.* (1996, 2001) used a combination of goal setting and measures in their research projects. This enabled goals to be fashioned individually for each child on the one hand, while on the other hand enabling results to be investigated more generally using a validated measure, so that comparisons could be drawn between groups of children receiving different amounts of intervention and groups of children undergoing different goal- and aim-setting procedures. Therapists were asked to identify their intervention objectives for each child and the dimensions in a validated evaluative measure in which change was expected as a result of those objectives. Children's motor functional status was classified according to the Gross Motor Function Classification System (GMFCS) (Palisano *et al.* 1997). In this classification children at level 1 walk without restrictions, children at level 2 walk without assistive devices, children at level 3 walk with assistive devices, children at level 4 have self-mobility with limitations, and children at level 5 are severely limited in self-mobility even with the use of assistive technology.

The one measure consistently used in all four studies was the GMFM-88 (Russell *et al.* 2002). This measure is a standardized observational instrument designed and validated to measure change in gross motor function over time in children with CP. The 88 items are ranged over five dimensions: Lying & Rolling; Sitting; Crawling & Kneeling; Standing; and Walking, Running & Jumping. Each item is scored on a four-point Likert scale.

As an example of the combination of goal-setting with the use of a validated measure, we look at the case of a 6-year-old girl who attended a special unit in a mainstream school. She had difficulties with concentration, and her behaviour tended to be labile. Her mother was rather fearful of letting her do things independently in case she hurt herself. Her father was away a lot. The girl was classified at level 4 on the GMFCS, had a developmental motor age of less than 8 months and a baseline score of 50% on the GMFM-88. She was restricted to floor mobility or used an electric wheelchair. When asked what her problems were she looked at her mother and said nothing. Both her mother and her teacher were primarily concerned with their backs. Her mother felt that it would be helpful if she could stand at the basin and toilet for washing and for donning and doffing her pants. Her teacher felt that it would be helpful if she could get in and out of her wheelchair independently. Her therapist was concerned with (1) a subluxating right hip, (2) a wheelchair that was inappropriate for the right hip and for getting in and out of, and (3) deterioration in her crawling. After discussion the following goals were set:

GOAL 1 (in three parts)
1. Sit on chair, pull to stand holding on to bar and maintain for 5 seconds.
2. Lift left hand off for 5 seconds and replace.
3. Lift right hand off for 5 seconds and replace.
Review in three weeks.

Baseline
Sits on chair and pulls to stand holding on to bar for 2 seconds = 13%.
Score
Part 1 = 20⅓% at review
Part 2 = 33⅓% at review
Part 3 = 33⅓% at review
Change in GMFM-88, Standing dimension.

GOAL 2
From the floor get into wheelchair.
Review in 4 weeks.
Baseline
Can pull up on to wheelchair seat on abdomen but cannot turn round to sit down = 50%.
Score
Turn half way round using arms = 25% at review.
Turn right round to sit on bottom = 25% at review.
Change in GMFM-88, Sitting dimension.

Review results
At 3 weeks review, Goal 1 was achieved 100%.
At 4 weeks review, Goal 2 was achieved 75%.
The final 25% of Goal 2 was still not achieved at 8 weeks re-review and was abandoned.

Other measures
Some other validated evaluative measures that might prove useful in combination with goal-setting are:
• The Gross Motor Performance Measure (GMPM) (Boyce *et al*. 1998) evaluates change in quality of gross motor function (alignment, coordination, dissociated movement, stability and weight shift) in children with CP from 5 months to 12 years. It takes between 45 and 60 minutes to administer by a qualified therapist trained in the use of the GMPM using the GMPM manual. It is obtainable from Dr William Boyce, School of Rehabilitation Therapy, Faculty of Health Sciences, Queen's University, Kingston KYL 3N6, Canada, for research purposes. It is currently being modified for clinical use by Virginia Wright at the *CanChild* Centre for Childhood Disability Research, Hamilton, Ontario, Canada.
• The WeeFIM (Msall *et al*. 1994) evaluates change in functional ability over time on a seven-point scale ranging from complete independence to total assistance required. Motor abilities are assessed in self-care, sphincter control, transfers and locomotion, and cognitive abilities are assessed in communication and social cognition. It takes 30 minutes to administer using a manual and is suitable for all children with developmental disabilities and a 'mental age' of less than 7 years. It is obtainable from State University of New York at Buffalo School of Medicine and Biomedical Sciences, The Centre for Functional Assessment Research, Uniform Data System for Medical Rehabilitation, 232 Parker Hall, Sunny South Campus, 3435 Main Street, Buffalo, New York 141214-3007, USA.
• Pediatric Evaluation of Disability Inventory (PEDI) (Haley *et al*. 1997), obtainable from

the Psychological Corporation, Footscray High Street, Sidcup, Kent DA14 5HP, England.
- The Movement Assessment Battery for Children (Movement ABC) (Henderson and Sugden 1992) evaluates movement problems (movement competence, manual dexterity, ball skills, static and dynamic balance) that can determine a child's participation and social adjustment at school. It can be used with children from 4 to 12 years of age and takes 30 minutes to administer by a therapist using the manual. It is published by the Psychological Corporation (address above).

Record keeping

Accurate documentation is necessary for goal setting and research. It enables recipients of services, professionals and managers to inform themselves retrospectively of the progress of events. In these days of increased litigation it is necessary for therapists to be able to show exactly what intervention has taken place and the reasons for it, and to document any foreseen and unforeseen consequences.

Audit

Clinical audit is a process by which the effectiveness of a clinical service can be repeatedly tested by critical observation and intervention using a systematic methodology, the results being fed back, leading directly to an improvement in practice (McLellan 1997).

Audit considers (1) clients, (2) service providers, and (3) interventions—all in one particular service.

Research

Research is the endeavour to discover new or collate old facts by scientific study of a subject or course of critical investigation (*Concise Oxford Dictionary*, cited by McLellan 1997).

Conclusion

Goal setting, measurement, audit and research all require a systematic approach and accuracy to be of any value. To date no randomized controlled trial has provided Sackett (1986) level 1 generalizable evidence to suggest that either quantitative changes ('whether' a child performs a motor function) or qualitative advances ('how' a child performs a motor function) have been the result of physical therapy intervention in children with CP. Therefore the identification of specific, measurable goals should be employed to log changes in individual children with cerebral palsy. The consistent use of collaborative goal setting will help to show whether a particular line of intervention can be shown to be helping a particular child, and whether outcome appears to be of greater benefit with one line of intervention than with another. Such action will help individual children, their families, teachers and therapists to make more informed decisions across intervention options.

REFERENCES

Bayley, N. (1993) *Bayley Scales of Infant Development (BSID II) Motor Scale Kit. 2nd Edn*. Sidcup, Kent: Psychological Corporation.

Bland, J.M., Altman, D.G. (1986) 'Statistical methods for assessing agreement between two methods of clinical measurement.' *Lancet*, **1**, 307–310.

Bower, E. (1997) 'The multiply handicapped child.' *In:* McLellan, D.L., Wilson, B. (Eds.) *The Handbook of Rehabilitation Studies*. Cambridge: Cambridge University Press, pp. 315–335.

Bower, E. (1999) 'Current techniques in physiotherapy for children with cerebral palsy.' *Current Paediatrics*, **9**, 79–83.

Bower, E., McLellan, D.L. (1992) 'Effects of increased exposure to physiotherapy on skill acquisition in children with cerebral palsy.' *Developmental Medicine and Child Neurology*, **34**, 25–39.

Bower, E., McLellan, D.L. (1994a) 'Assessing motor skill acquisition in four centres for the treatment of children with cerebral palsy.' *Developmental Medicine and Child Neurology*, **36**, 902–909.

Bower, E., McLellan, D.L. (1994b) 'Evaluating therapy in cerebral palsy.' *Child: Care, Health and Development*, **20**, 409–419.

Bower, E., McLellan, D.L. (1994c) 'Measuring motor goals in children with cerebral palsy.' *Clinical Rehabilitation*, **8**, 198–206.

Bower, E., McLellan, D.L., Arney, J., Campbell, M.J. (1996) 'A randomised controlled trial of different intensities of physiotherapy and different goal setting procedures in 44 children with cerebral palsy.' *Developmental Medicine and Child Neurology*, **38**, 226–238.

Bower, E., Michell, D.M., Burnett, M., Campbell, M.J., McLellan, D.L. (2001) 'Randomised controlled trial of physiotherapy in 56 children with cerebral palsy followed for 18 months.' *Developmental Medicine and Child Neurology*, **43**, 4–25.

Boyce, W., Gowland, C., Rosenbaum, P., Hardy, S., Lane, M., Plews, N., Goldsmith, C., Russell, D., Wright. V., Potter, S., Harding, D. (1998) *Gross Motor Performance Measure Manual*. Kingston, Ontario: Queen's University School of Rehabilitation Therapy.

Cogher, L., Savage, E., Smith, M.F. (1992) *Cerebral Palsy. The Child and Young Person*. London: Chapman Hall Medical.

Collis, E. (1947) *A Way of Life for the Handicapped Child*. London. Faber & Faber.

Cotton, E. (1980) *The Basic Motor Pattern*. London: The Spastics Society.

Finnie, N.R. (1997) *Handling the Young Child with Cerebral Palsy at Home*. London: Butterworth, Heinemann.

Folio, R.M., Fewell, R.R. (2000) *Peabody Development Motor Scales, 2nd Edn. (PDMS-2.)* Sidcup, Kent: Psychological Corporation.

Gowland, C., King, G., King, S., Low, M., Lette, L., MacKinnon, L., Rosenbaum, P., Russell, D. (1991) *Review of Selected Measures in Neurodevelopmental Rehabilitation – a Rational Approach for Selecting Clinical Measures – Research Report 91–92*. Ontario: Neurodevelopmental Clinical Research Unit, Chedoke-McMaster Hospitals.

Greenhough, W.T., Black, J.E., Wallace, C.S. (1987) 'Experience and brain development.' *Child Development*, **58**, 539–559.

Haley, S.M., Coster, W.J., Ludlow, L.H., Haltiwanger, J.T., Andrellos, P.J. (1992) *Pediatric Evaluation of Disability Inventory (PEDI) Development, Standardisation and Administration Manual*. Sidcup, Kent: Psychological Corporation.

Henderson, S.E., Sugden, D.A. (1992) *Movement Assessment Battery for Children (Movement ABC)*. Sidcup, Kent: Psychological Corporation.

Herbert, M. (1987) *Behavioural Treatment of Children with Problems. A Practical Manual. 2nd Edn.* London: Academic Press, Harcourt Brace.

Illingworth, R.S., Lister, J. (1964) 'The critical or sensitive period, with special reference to certain 'feeding problems' in infants and children.' *Journal of Pediatrics*, **65**, 839–848.

Kirschner, B., Guyatt, G. (1985) 'A methodological framework for assessing health indices.' *Journal of Chronic Disease*, **38**, 27–36.

McGraw, M. (1943) *The Neuromuscular Maturation of the Human Infant*. New York. Columbia University Press. (Republished as *Classics in Developmental Medicine No. 4*. London: Mac Keith Press, 1990.)

McLellan, D.L. (1997) 'Introduction to rehabilitation.' *In:* McLellan, D.L., Wilson, B. (Eds.) *The Handbook of Rehabilitation Studies*. Cambridge: Cambridge University Press, pp. 14–15.

Msall, M.E., Di Gandio, K., Duffy, L.C. (1994) 'WeeFIM: Normative sample of an instrument for tracking functional independence in children.' *Clinical Pediatrics*, **33**, 431–438.

O'Dwyer, N., Neilson, P., Nash, J. (1989) 'Mechanisms of muscle growth related to muscle contracture in cerebral palsy.' *Developmental Medicine and Child Neurology*, **3**, 1543–1552.

Palisano, R., Rosenbaum, P., Walter, S., Russell, D., Wood, E., Galuppi, B. (1997) 'Development and reliability of a system to classify gross motor function in children with cerebral palsy.' *Developmental Medicine and Child Neurology*, **39**, 214–223.

Rosenbaum, P., Walter, S.D., Hanna, S.E., Palisano, R.J., Russell, D.J., Raina, P., Wood. E., Bartlett, D.J., Galuppi, B.E. (2002) 'Prognosis for gross motor function in cerebral palsy.' *Journal of the American Medical Association*, **288**, 1357–1363.

Russell, D., Rosenbaum, P., Gowland, C., Hardy, S., Lane M., Plews N., McGavin H., Cadman, D., Jars, S. (1993) *The Gross Motor Function Measure, 2nd Edn.* Toronto: Hugh Macmillan Rehabilitation Center, McMaster University.

Russell, D.J., Rosenbaum, P.L., Avery, L.M., Lane, M. (2002) *Gross Motor Function Measure (GMFM-66 and GMFM-88) User's Manual. Clinics in Developmental Medicine No. 159.* London: Mac Keith Press.

Sackett, D.L. (1986) 'Rules of evidence and clinical recommendations on the use of antithrombic agents.' *Chest*, **89**, 25–35.

Wade, D. (1992) *Measurement in Neurological Rehabilitation*. Oxford: Oxford University Press.

WHO (2002) *International Classification of Function, Disability and Health. ICIDH-2.* Geneva: World Health Organization.

5

A PHYSIOTHERAPY PERSPECTIVE ON ASSESSMENT AND OUTCOME MEASUREMENT OF CHILDREN WITH CEREBRAL PALSY

Roslyn N. Boyd

The aim of any physiotherapy programme for children with cerebral palsy (CP) is to enable them to achieve their optimal potential by reducing the degree of disability and promoting participation in a daily social context. Inherent in a successful management programme is a rational approach to assessment and outcome measurement. This can be undertaken only with knowledge of typical performance, the expected natural history, possible response to various interventions and an ability to elicit optimal performance from the child being assessed. Within the multidisciplinary team physiotherapists play an important role in the assessment of children with CP. They have a unique background in the observation of movement, and are gaining advanced knowledge in biomechanics and the neurosciences to help understand the pathophysiology underlying the condition. They work closely with other team members such as paediatric orthopaedic surgeons, neurologists, rehabilitation specialists, paediatricians, biomechanists, occupational therapists, speech therapists and orthotists to define goals, select treatment options and monitor the time course of the motor disorder. Paediatric physiotherapists are trained to assess the quality of movement, and a background in biomechanics provides an important supplement to quantify motor performance, functional abilities and activity limitations. Measures of the pathophysiology underlying motor performance are less available to them. Physiotherapists are realizing more than ever the need to take account of the whole child, rather than focusing purely on gross motor skills and ambulation, by measuring fine motor skills, occupational performance and societal participation.

The focus of this chapter will be on the rationales for physiotherapy approaches to assessment of the child with CP, and the selection and use of assessment tools for identifying appropriate intervention strategies, monitoring management and measuring outcome.

High tech, low tech, no tech

Depending on their work setting, paediatric physiotherapists use a wide range of assessments some requiring sophisticated instrumentation and expertise ('high tech'), some needing substantially less training and/or equipment ('low tech') and others that are more experience based ('no tech'). There are many assessments and outcome measures that can be used by a clinician in a gait analysis laboratory or by a researcher conducting clinical trials that may not be practical or indeed relevant for clinicians in the community. Some 'high tech' tools are expensive, time consuming, labour intensive and not readily available, and thus are geared more to a specialized clinical center or a research setting. Other, 'low tech', tools are less costly, readily available and useful in a variety of settings. More important than any research or clinical tool is our ability to interpret the findings of these tests, to observe movement, elicit optimal performance, and assess family and child dynamics. These are our 'no tech tools', the skills we have learned from our training and through developing our own clinical reasoning and practice.

Practical clinical tools are often included in the evaluation of outcomes in research protocols, but many of the instrumented measures required to measure more precise or subtle increments of change are not available to the clinician. A growing number of research and clinical measures are available for both the upper and lower limbs of children with CP that span all domains of the International Classification of Functioning, Disability and Health (ICF: WHO 2001). A differentiation into 'high tech' and 'low tech' tools emphasizes our need to extrapolate what we have learned from the 'high tech' tools and apply these principles to assessment and outcome measurement in the clinical setting with 'low tech' tools (Boyd and Hayes 2001b).

Many clinicians in the community might consider the use of quantitative assessment tools and outcome measures to be geared purely to a research setting. With the ever-growing need to justify funding for therapy for children with disabilities and the need to measure the effectiveness of clinical practice it is perhaps more important than ever for clinicians to contribute to the outcome measurement process. There are several excellent websites and initiatives that have made outcome measures more accessible to the clinician [e.g. CanChild, http://canchild.interlynx.net; American Physical Therapy Association (APTA), www.apta.org]. New funding initiatives supported by efficacy or effectiveness data may enable existing programmes to be continued or increased amounts of therapy to be provided; however, the outcomes need to be measured in a way that can continue to justify that ongoing funding. Increasingly we need to use a standard set of assessments that have been shown to be meaningful, have repeatability, validity, and utility for use in the clinical setting.

Another important reason for the use of assessment and outcome measures is that children and their parents want to know how they performed: did they get faster, could they walk further than last time in their 10 minute walking test, what was their score on the Gross Motor Function Measure (GMFM) last year, are they steadily improving and holding their own in the presence of rapid growth? As physiotherapists we often emphasize how we have reduced their spasticity or improved their alignment, and while these factors may be relevant to us they may not be meaningful or motivating to the child. For example, all children with congenital hemiplegia will walk (usually independently) but use of their impaired upper limbs may impact more on their functional independence, education and vocational aspirations. The use of disablement models such as the ICF encourages physiotherapists to assess children across a spectrum of outcomes of interest to both the child and the clinician/researcher.

Rationales for assessment

NATURAL HISTORY

Two major factors influencing the rationale for assessment are an understanding of the natural history of the movement disorder and the need for standardized serial or longitudinal assessments rather than single measures. The 'natural' history of the musculoskeletal pathology in children with CP reflects gradual progression of the musculoskeletal pathology over time (Rang 1990; see also Chapter 8). Physiotherapists need to have a detailed knowledge of the natural progression of the spastic motor disorders to assess the child with respect to the anticipated change in motor function. Physiotherapists should educate parents about what to expect; why some muscles may become overactive, increasingly stiff or short especially during periods of rapid growth; and why as children approach adolescence there may be an increasing tendency to muscle contracture, bony malalignment and weakness in the antigravity muscles.

A good example of the importance of understanding natural history is recognition of the need for monitoring of hip displacement in children with bilateral spastic CP. Hip dislocation is frequently preventable, but as lateral hip displacement may be clinically silent it can be monitored effectively only by six-monthly serial pelvic radiographs, using standardized positioning and careful measurement (Scrutton and Baird 1997, Scrutton et al. 2001, Dobson et al. 2002, Parrott et al. 2002).

The second important factor in monitoring natural history is the limitation of single data point assessments in determining the prognosis. For example, recent studies have shown that sequential monitoring of generalized movements of preterm infants may be more predictive of motor outcome than individual assessments (Cioni et al. 1997, Hadders-Algra et al. 1997, Lacey and Henderson-Smart 1998, Prechtl 2001). An even clearer indication of prognosis of motor outcome may be seen by determining change in a motor score in response to changes in environmental factors. Assessment of a young infant with motor delay at 14 weeks corrected age can be influenced by the predominant practice that the child has experienced. If the infant is a predominantly supine sleeping baby and has spent only limited periods of time in prone then motor assessment of prone skills and the overall score on the Movement Assessment of Infants (MAI, Swanson et al. 1992) will be influenced negatively. The change in the MAI score after a two-week period of prone experience may be more predictive of motor outcome and the infant's adaptation to environmental changes than the original MAI score.

A BIOMECHANICAL LANGUAGE

In a multidisciplinary team a biomechanical language is a common framework that can be understood by all team members and provides a quantitative approach. There are many excellent texts that explain a biomechanical approach to gait evaluation (e.g. Sutherland et al. 1988, Gage 1992, Perry 1992). These seminal texts describe the important biomechanical principles of normal and pathological gait and are important reading for every clinician working with children with CP.

In a 'high tech' gait analysis laboratory, a biomechanical language is used to assess children and monitor outcome. Families may also find a description of function in simple biomechanical terms far easier to understand than much of the medical terminology we use. They may find it easier to understand muscle function as 'overactivity or stiffness' rather than 'spasticity or hypertonia'. There is still considerable controversy amongst clinicians and researchers about spasticity management in children with CP because of the lack of clear definitions (Boyd and Ada 2001, Sanger *et al.* 2003). A more 'low tech' approach could be undertaken by assessing gait and postural patterns through systematic observation, performing a comprehensive orthopaedic examination and using a biomechanical approach to prescribing and tuning orthoses based on descriptions such as Perry's ankle rockers (Perry 1992). Clinicians in the community can use the lessons learnt from instrumented gait analysis to improve their clinical reasoning, yet must realize the limitations and assumptions underlying 'low tech' information.

The Physicians Rating Scale (PRS) as developed by Koman *et al.* (1994), modified initially by Corry *et al.* (1998) then modified further as the Observational Gait Scale (OGS, Boyd and Graham 1999) is a simple 'low tech' tool designed for assessment of younger children with predominantly sagittal plane gait deviations who are considered too small or non-compliant for three-dimensional gait analysis (3DGA). The OGS has been shown to have good reliability in the sagittal plane and has recently been validated against instrumented gait analysis, the 'gold standard' (Mackie *et al.* 2003). The authors recognize the limitations of the OGS in the coronal and transverse planes, and clinicians should consider referral for instrumented gait analysis where complex gait deviations exist.

Instrumented gait analysis should be the assessment of choice in ambulant children for whom multiple-level surgeries, irreversible surgery (selective dorsal rhizotomy, SDR) or other invasive, expensive options (intrathecal baclofen, ITB) are considered. Instrumented 3DGA is an important tool for quantifying the gait deviations in all three planes, delineating primary gait deviations due to the initial pathology, secondary compensations due to growth and maturation from tertiary gait deviations (voluntary compensations to overcome the limitations of the primary and secondary problems) (Gage 1992). To obtain an accurate 3DGA the child must be at least 1.0 m tall, weigh more than 20 kg (for accurate kinetics) and be able to cooperate (4 years and older). When assessing children outside these limits the clinician can still utilize biomechanical principles learnt in the gait laboratory for visual observation of gait. Initially they should classify the typical gait pattern from visual observation or from slow-motion video recordings (Boyd and Graham 1997, 1999; Rodda and Graham 2001), then consider the relative contribution of the positive and negative features of the upper motor neuron syndrome to the gait pattern (Boyd and Graham 1999, Boyd and Ada 2001). Figure 5.1 gives a good example of the integration of 'low tech' information gained by observation of gait, linked to an understanding of 3DGA, 'high tech' information.

Direct correlation between static and dynamic measures of lower-extremity range of motion is poor in children with CP and control populations (McMulkin *et al.* 2000). Inconsistencies in range of motion measures between the clinical examination and instrumented motion analysis may be a result of changes in muscle tone, strength, balance and motor control during gait, or may be a result of differences in angle definitions used in each situation (Ounpuu *et al.* 2001). Neither of these measures should be discounted, but dynamic movement abnormalities should take precedence over muscle lengths examined clinically

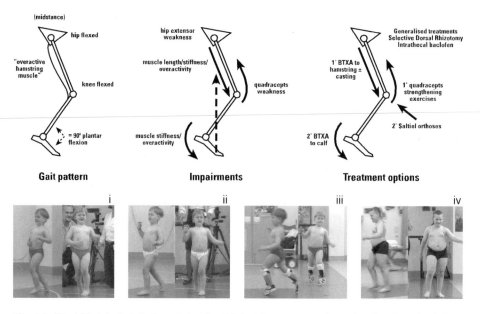

Fig. 5.1. *(Top)* Model of clinical reasoning for child with apparent equines, showing (i) sagittal plane alignment of gait pattern in mid-stance; (ii) possible relative contribution of impairments with ground reaction force vector (dotted arrow); (iii) primary and secondary treatment options.

(Bottom) Boy with spastic diplegia with apparent equinus gait and GMFCS level II. Note sagittal and coronal view of gait pattern at (i) 16 months of age; (ii) 24 months after a programme of intramuscular injections of botulinum toxin A (BTX-A) to the hamstrings supplemented by two weeks of long leg serial plasters; (iii) 4 years of age after two episodes of BTX-A, use of ground-reaction ankle–foot orthoses and gait training; and (iv) 10 years of age after a programme of spasticity management with intrathecal baclofen and single-event multiple-level surgery combined with physiotherapy and appropriate orthoses.

when making treatment recommendations. In addition to understanding the definitions of gait measures taken and the assumptions of models used in 3DGA, one should be careful to obtain the most accurate clinical measures in order to assign probable causes to gait deviations seen on 3DGA.

EVIDENCE-BASED PRACTICE

A growing influence on clinical practice is the use of evidence-based medicine (EBM) (Sackett *et al*. 2001). An EBM approach in measuring outcomes and reviewing physiotherapy trials is now readily available for the clinician on websites [Treatment Outcomes committee of the American Academy of Cerebral Palsy and Developmental Medicine (AACPDM) website, http://www.aacpdm.org/committees/treatmentoutcomes.html; Physiotherapy Evidence Database (PEDro) website, www.pedro.fhs.usyd.edu.au] and in systematic reviews of treatment options (Boyd and Hayes 2001a, Boyd *et al*. 2001b, McLaughlin *et al*. 2002). The use of classification systems such as the Gross Motor Function Classification System, (GMFCS, Palisano *et al*. 1997) and the Winters and Gage classification of gait in hemiplegia (Winters *et al*. 1987) can help in relating the findings of research trials to children in the clinic. Summaries of outcome measures are now available (American Physical Therapy Association 2001, Law *et al.* 2001) that provide detailed information on the reliability, validity, and responsiveness of commonly used assessment tools. It is hoped that in the future a link will be established between databases of outcome measures and evidence-based databases of high-quality studies using these tools.

TYPES OF MEASUREMENT TOOLS

Kirshner and Guyatt (1985) have classified health measurement instruments by their ability to (1) discriminate between individuals, (2) predict future status, and (3) evaluate change and function over time or after treatment. Preliminary assessment of children with CP encourages clinicians to use measures that discriminate between individuals in order to define the child amongst his peer group and to compare that child with other children defined in the literature, for example by the GMFCS (Palisano *et al.* 1997) or the Pediatric Evaluation of Disability Inventory (PEDI, Haley *et al.* 1991). A predictive measure is one that can usefully estimate future function based on current performance, such as the GMFCS. Besides its discriminative capabilities, current GMFCS classification system categorizations can also be used to predict future Gross Motor Function Measure scores using gross motor curves developed from extensive cross-sectional and longitudinal data (Rosenbaum *et al.* 2002).

The third purpose of a clinical measure is as an evaluative tool to measure the presence or amount of change in clinical parameter over time (Kirschner and Guyatt 1985). For example, several clinical tools and instrumented measures are available for the measurement of energy consumption in children with CP. Clinical tools such as the Energy Expenditure Index (EEI, Rose *et al.* 1991) and Physiological Cost Index (PCI, Butler *et al.* 1984) may have limited usefulness due to the variability of heart rate in most young children whether healthy or disabled (Boyd *et al.* 1999a). Instrumented measures that evaluate oxygen consumption and cost, such as the Cosmed K4 (Cosmed, Italy), have significant measurement error (13% of the mean in able-bodied children) making the range needed to show clinical changes (change expected to be due to a treatment rather than to day-to-day variability) quite large (18% in able-bodied children, 22% in able-bodied adults) and possibly even greater in children with CP (Boyd *et al.* 1999b). The high variability in testing of energy consumption using the PCI, even in the laboratory highlights its probable limited usefulness in the community setting. However, a 10-minute walk on a circular walking track using a heart-rate monitor and step monitor (pedometer) can provide other helpful information on distance walked, endurance, and stability of heart rate in what may be a submaximal test for marginal ambulators (Boyd *et al.* 1999b). This information may be a more useful predictor in evaluating a child's ability to cope with a programme of multiple-level surgery and rehabilitation after surgery.

MEASUREMENT PROPERTIES OF INSTRUMENTS

Reports of measurement properties of clinical assessments need to include information on how much change must occur to be of mathematical (greater than the standard error of measurement) and functional relevance, as this is the bottom line for clinicians. They need to know the acceptable variability between experienced raters in standardized conditions

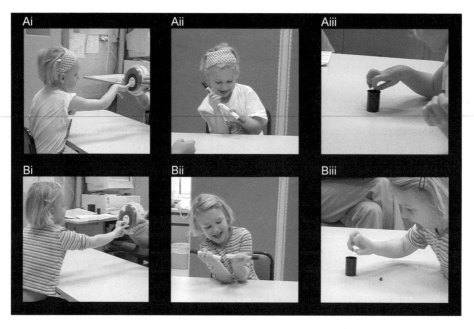

Fig. 5.2. Five-year-old girl with right hemiplegia at baseline (Ai–Aiii) and at three weeks after intramuscular injections of botulinum toxin A to the spastic forearm muscles (Bi–Biii). Note changes in biomechanical alignment in reaching to a target (i), improved supination in a two-pen tapping task (ii), and improved wrist and elbow extension and supination in fine grasp (iii).

as opposed to inexperienced raters. One of the greatest difficulties for physiotherapists in both the research and clinical setting is whether an evaluative measurement tool will be responsive enough to measure change due to that treatment in the group being studied. 'Natural' history studies can assist in determining expected change with usual clinical practice. Russell *et al.* (1993) reported increases of 6% per year with the GMFM in children with diplegia, and 4% per year in children with quadriplegia. However, for high-functioning children with hemiplegia (GMFCS levels I and II), there may be a ceiling effect as the baseline score offers limited range for improvement (Love *et al.* 2001). It may be more appropriate to set 'goal areas' on the GMFM a priori for outcome measurement that are the aims of the treatment or use proportional change of measures to monitor outcome (Blair *et al.* 2001). The limited abilities and potential for improvement in children with severe quadriplegia (GMFCS level V) means that a 'floor effect' may also exist where there is poor sensitivity in severely affected children (Boyd *et al.* 2001a). Rasch scaling of the GMFM has improved the efficiency and scaling of GMFM scores and may help reduce ceiling effects (Russell *et al.* 2000).

The measurement properties of tools might also limit the responsiveness of the measure to certain treatments as well as certain patient subgroups (Preston and Colman 2000). The PEDI has two response categories (unable/capable of performing items in most situations) (Haley *et al.* 1991), thus ignoring biomechanical changes (Fig. 5.2). For children with hemiplegia, measurement on the Self Care domain of the PEDI could be limited as they might be able to perform the task in an awkward manner one-handed prior to intra-muscular injections of botulinum toxin A (BTX-A) and upper-limb training, but might then perform this more efficiently with both hands after training. It is therefore important to consider whether we measure what we aim to train. The Melbourne Unilateral Upper-Limb Assessment (MUL) is a reliable measure of impaired arm function that quantifies biome-chanical changes after BTX-A upper-limb training (Randall *et al.* 2001). In contrast, the Assisting Hand Assessment (AHA) quantifies bilateral motor skillsin children with uni-lateral upper-limb impairments (Kramlinde-Sundholm and Eliasson 2003). The PEDI may not be sensitive to these changes in upper-limb motor behaviour. Researchers need to use all their clinical knowledge in designing meaningful clinical trials with appropriate and mean-ingful outcome measures with validity, reliability and responsiveness set in a child-oriented context.

Most importantly, the assessment procedure should be meaningful and fun for the child to participate in as testing protocols that lack relevance and are tedious will not obtain an optimal performance. Much of the success of optimal performance lies with the clinician to presenting the tasks in a language understood by the child, with relevance to their concept of their motor disorder and based on sound rationales with empirical evidence.

AN ASSESSMENT MODEL FOR THE MOTOR DISORDER IN CHILDREN WITH CP
1. Define the patient problem
If the child is able to tell you, first find out how they define their problems/difficulties, then ask the parents/carers. Next the clinician needs to define their perception of the child's and family's problems based on the information they have been given (referral letter, their observations of the child's posture and movement skills). The principles of evidence-based practice can then help in framing a clinically meaningful question (Sackett *et al.* 2001).

2. Classify overall functional status
In order to define how the child compares with those in the research literature it is helpful to classify her/him according to the GMFCS (Palisano *et al.* 1997). Recently, gross motor curves have been developed for children at each level by assessing their GMFM scores at different ages (Rosenbaum *et al.* 2002). This may be helpful for the therapist and the parent in devising realistic goals for mobility/functional independence.

3. Confirm pathophysiology
For this model I will assume that the family has been given a diagnosis of CP for their child (Badawi *et al.* 1998). While undertaking the motor assessment, consider the etiology of the condition. For instance, is the original brain lesion one of the following: motor cortex lesion leading to spasticity or dystonia; basal ganglia lesion leading to rigidity/dyskinesia; cerebellar lesion leading to ataxia; or a genetic disorder? Consider the type of tone or movement abnormality, *i.e.* spasticity, dystonia, rigidity or mixed types (Sanger *et al.* 2003), athetosis or ataxia, and the topography, *i.e.* monoplegia, hemiplegia, diplegia, triplegia, quadriplegia (Gage 1992).

4. Review current medical status and relevant medical history
Consider current general health and well being, including comorbidity such as epilepsy, mental retardation, malnutrition and behavior and how they impact on motor performance. For example, poor oral motor function or impaired nutrition may lead to weakness, fatigue or poor initiation of motor tasks.

5. Measure current performance for the motor task(s) of greatest concern to child and family
Use a measurement tool considered to be relevant, reliable, valid and appropriate for the setting. In the absence of a measurement tool the clinician can video the child performing the task, initially unassisted or barefoot, then with appropriate caregiver assistance, and use of gait aids and orthoses, then undertake a task analysis (Gentile 1987).

6. Classify the child's postural and gait patterns
Children with spastic type CP have been recognized as having postural patterns that evolve over time and may be distinct in terms of severity and maturation of motor abilities. In the non- ambulant or pre-ambulatory child consider the presence of scissoring hip postures in stepping when supported, posture in long sitting (*e.g.* presence of sacral sitting indicates short hamstrings), typical sitting and lying postures (presence of hip flexion with adduction or abduction, windswept hips, preferential head turning or trunk rotation).

For the child who ambulates take account of alignment of the lower limbs in the sagittal plane during walking. Several authors have presented sagittal plane biomechanical classification of gait in diplegia (Sutherland and Davids 1993, Boyd and Graham 1999, Rodda and Graham 2001). As with all classification systems it is not yet known how stable these patterns will be over time with the natural history of the condition or in response to the intervention. For children with problems in the coronal plane, consider limb-length discrepancies (true or apparent) and asymmetries. In the transverse plane, consider bony torsion contributing to lever-arm disease such as femoral anteversion, tibial torsion or foot malalignment (Gage 1992, Ruwe *et al*. 1992).

For the child with hemiplegia, a kinematic classification system exists for gait patterns I to IV based on 3DGA (Winters *et al*. 1987) that is typically used to guide treatment recommendations (Novacheck 2001). This classification enables physiotherapists to have a better understanding of the relationships between ankle, knee and hip involvement with increasing severity from grades I to IV. In a similar way, there may be increasing complexity with severity (distal to proximal) in the upper limb.

In both the lower and upper limbs, motor patterns may vary over time and in response to treatment. Motion restrictions may occur faster in some muscles than others, with progressive muscle stiffness leading to muscle contracture termed the 'biological clock' (Boyd and Graham 1997). Recognition of those muscles that are more overactive than others can help predict impending motor dysfunction and deformity (Boyd and Graham 1997).

7. Determine the relative contribution of various impairments
Careful measurement of the positive features (spasticity, muscle contracture, dystonia) and

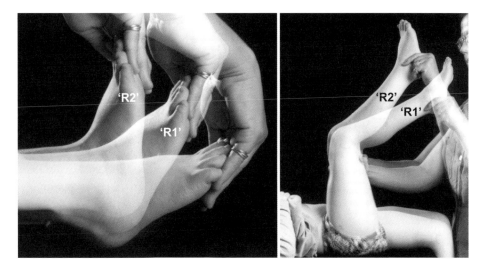

Fig. 5.3. Assessments of dynamic range of motion 'R1' at the ankle and knee as conducted by the author's modification of the Tardieu scale (Tardieu *et al.* 1954). 'R2' is the slow passive range of motion (conducted at Tardieu velocity V1). 'R1' is the fast velocity movement of the ankle through full available range of motion to determine the point of 'catch' in the range of motion (Tardieu velocity V3). The angle at which the muscle reaction ('catch' or 'R1') occurs is measured by goniometry. (a) the Tardieu measure is performed at the ankle to test the gastrocnemius with the knee extended. (b) The Tardieu measure is performed for the hamstring muscles with the hip flexed to 90° and the opposite hip extended. (Reprinted by permission from Boyd and Graham 1999.)

negative features (weakness, loss of selective motor control) of the upper motor neuron syndrome at each level (hips, knees, ankles, shoulder, elbow, wrist, trunk) can indicate the relative contribution of impairments to motor patterns in different tasks (Boyd and Ada 2001).

Assessment of positive impairments. Careful clinical examination of the slow passive range of motion limit or 'R2' at (Tardieu velocity V1) using 'notable' or maximal force can quantify muscle length at each level (Tardieu *et al.* 1954, Boyd and Graham 1999). If one is assessing spasticity, this is then compared to the fast velocity (V3) range of motion, attempting to use the same force and consistent speed throughout the motion, to determine the spastic 'catch' angle defined as 'R1'. Perhaps more important than these individual measures is the difference between 'R2' and 'R1' (Fig. 5.3). A larger difference indicates a larger reflexive component (spasticity), whereas a smaller difference may indicate greater muscle contracture than spasticity. These relationships should then be considered alongside the classification of the sagittal gait pattern in deciding which levels to treat (hip, knee, ankle) with which management options (Boyd and Graham 1999). In general, reliability of goniometric measurement can be improved by standardizing the conditions of testing, careful consideration of the proximal and distal segments to be measured and their reference criteria, use of standardized 'notable or maximum' force, use of single degree increments on the goniometer, and employing the same experienced examiner for each examination (Stuberg *et al.* 1988, Eliasziw *et al.* 1994, McDowell *et al.* 2001).

Assessment of negative impairments. The clinician must also take account of the negative impairments at each level, including strength and selective motor control. Some normative isometric strength data for able-bodied children and children with CP are available (Wiley and Damiano 1998); however, the clinician must standardize the testing protocol, consider the repeatability of the maximum voluntary contraction and the differences in body mass and limb length for comparison over time or between subjects. Assessments of selective motor control are few and confined to comparison of clinical assessment of ability to activate the dorsiflexors to a visual cue called the 'selective motor control test' (Boyd and Graham 1999) and postural balance of the dorsiflexors of the foot in the 'confusion test' (Davids *et al.* 1993). More tests of dexterity related to functional tasks in the upper and lower limbs in children with CP are needed.

8. Measuring functional attainment (activity limitation), participation in society and health-related quality of life

Many new assessment measures have been developed that quantify function and participation in children with CP, with quality of life measures lagging somewhat behind. Choices among these will depend on the age of the child, the functional status, the goal of the assessment or intervention, and the patient's priorities for seeking care (Boyd and Hayes 2001b). In general, assessments of participation are geared to measurement of performance in everyday settings. They are frequently difficult to measure objectively, and performance is often based on self-report or parent report. There is an increasing emphasis on determining what it is that children do in the 'real world'. The PEDI is a global measure of activity and participation useful in comparing the child to a normative sample (Haley *et al.* 1991). It provides a useful context for determining current performance and the amount of caregiver assistance prior to setting individualized goals. The clinician might use measures of participation and societal involvement at the beginning of a programme or at regular intervals (annually) to ensure that management programmes are relevant to the child in her/his environment (*e.g.* the Canadian Occupational Performance Measure, Law *et al.* 1994; the Goal Attainment Scale, Maloney *et al.* 1978). There are several measures developed to assess children's health-related quality of life on a generic scale. To date there are no published condition-specific tools of health-related quality of life for children with CP.

9. Adverse events and unintended effects

Physiotherapists, by virtue of their often more frequent contact with children and their families, should be mindful of unintended or unexpected effects due to a treatment as only careful clinical observation can highlight some previously unreported effects, such as incontinence in children after BTX-A injections (Boyd *et al.* 1996). They need to work closely with other team members to monitor and report any adverse events in clinical practice or formal trials (Boyd *et al.* 1999b, Baker *et al.* 2002).

The future

The paediatric physiotherapist in the community needs to select a standard set of measurement tools that are reliable and meaningful, taking account of the full spectrum of the disablement model from impairment and function through to participation, and utilizing sound biomechanical principles. While 'high tech' tools such as instrumented gait analysis and brain imaging will become increasingly sophisticated and guide us as to the pathophysiology underlying conditions, we will still rely to a large extent in many clinical settings on our 'low tech' and 'no tech' clinical tools. With the increasing availability of databases of outcome measures and evidence for treatment based on those measures it may soon become possible for clinicians to share data in large pooled samples so that clinically relevant questions can be answered. Randomized controlled clinical trials may provide efficacy for new treatments in small homogeneous samples, but an understanding of the effect on natural history of the motor disorder can be answered only across large population-based studies from CP registers. Clinicians and researchers must increasingly take account of disablement models to consider measurement not only of impairments and activity limitations but also of participation in society and health-related quality of life.

REFERENCES

American Physical Therapy Association (2001) 'Guide to Physical Therapist Practice. 2nd Edn.' *Physical Therapy*, **81**, 9–746.

Badawi, N.L., Watson, L., Petterson, B., Blair, E., Slee, J., Haan, E, Stanley, F.J. (1998) 'What constitutes cerebral palsy?' *Developmental Medicine and Child Neurology*, **40**, 520–527.

Baker, R., Jasinski, M., Maciag-Tymecka, I, Michalowska-Mrozek, J., Bonikowski, M., Carr, L., MacLean, J., Lin, J-P., Lynch, B., Theologis, T., Wendorff, J., Eunson, P., Cosgrove, A. (2002) 'Botulinum toxin treatment of spasticity in diplegic cerebral palsy: a randomized, double-blind, placebo-controlled, dose-ranging study.' *Developmental Medicine and Child Neurology*, **44**, 666–675.

Blair, E.M., Love, S.C., Valentine, J.P. (2001) 'Proportional change: an additional method of reporting technical and functional outcomes following clinical interventions.' *European Journal of Neurology*, **8**, Suppl. 5, 178–182.

Boyd, R., Bach, T., Morris, M., Imms, C., Johnson, L.., Graham, H.K., Syngeniotis, A., Abbott, D., Jackson, G. (2002) 'A randomized trial of botulinum toxin A and upper limb training—a functional MRI study.' *Developmental Medicine and Child Neurology*, **44**, Suppl. 91, 9. *(Abstract.)*

Boyd, R.N., Ada, L. (2001) 'Physiotherapy management of spasticity in adults and children with motor disability.' *In:* Barnes, M., Johnson, G. (Eds.) *Clinical Management of Spasticity.* Cambridge: Cambridge University Press, pp. 96–121.

Boyd, R.N., Graham, H.K. (1997) 'Botulinum toxin A in the management of children with cerebral palsy – indications and outcome.' *European Journal of Neurology*, **4**, Suppl. 2, 15–22.

Boyd, R.N., Graham, H.K. (1999) 'Objective clinical measures in the use of botulinum toxin A in the management of cerebral palsy.' *European Journal of Neurology*, **6**, Suppl. 4, S23–S36.

Boyd, R.N., Hayes, R. (2001a) 'Current evidence for botulinum toxin A in management of cerebral palsy – a systematic review.' *European Journal of Neurology*, **8**, Suppl. 5, 1–20.

Boyd, R.N., Hayes, R. (2001b) 'Outcome measures in cerebral palsy using an ICIDH-2 approach.' *European Journal of Neurology*, **8**, Suppl. 5, 167–177.

Boyd, R.N., Britton, T.C., Robinson, R.O., Borzyskowski, M. (1996) 'Transient urinary incontinence after botulinum toxin A.' *Lancet*, **348**, 481–482.

Boyd, R.N., Fatone, S., Rodda, J., Olesch, C., Starr, R., Cullis, E., Gallagher, D., Carlin, J.B., Nattrass, G.R., Graham, H.K. (1999a) 'High- or low-technology measurements of energy expenditure in clinical gait analysis?' *Developmental Medicine and Child Neurology*, **41**, 676–682.

Boyd, R.N., Graham, J., Nattrass, G., Graham, H.K. (1999b) 'Medium term outcomes and risk factor analysis in the use of botulinum toxin A in the management of cerebral palsy.' *European Journal of Neurology*, **6**, Suppl. 4, S37–S46.

Boyd, R.N., Dobson, F., Parrott, J., Love, S., Oates, J., Larsen, A., Burchall, G., Chondros, P., Carlin, J., Nattrass, G.R., Graham, H.K. (2001a) 'The effect of botulinum toxin A and a variable hip abduction orthosis on gross motor function: a randomised controlled trial.' *European Journal of Neurology*, **8**, Suppl. 5, 109–119.

Boyd, R.N., Morri, M., Graham, H.K. (2001b) 'A systematic review of management of the upper limb in children with cerebral palsy.' *European Journal of Neurology*, **8**, Suppl. 5, 150–166.

Butler, P., Engelbrecht, M., Major, R.E., Tait, J.H., Stallard, J., Patrick, J.H. (1984) 'Physiological cost index of walking for normal children and its use as an indicator of physical handicap/' *Developmental Medicine and Child Neurology*, **26**, 607–612.

Cioni, G., Prechtl, H.F., Ferrari, F., Paolicelli, P.B., Einspieler, C., Roversi, M.F. (1997) 'Which better predicts later outcome in full term infants: quality of general movements or neurological examination?' *Early Human Development*, **50**, 71–85.

Corry, I.S., Cosgrove, A.P., Duffy, C.M., McNeill, S., Taylor, T.C., Graham, H.K. (1998) 'Botulinum toxin A compared with stretching casts in the treatment of spastic equinus: a randomized prospective trial.' *Journal of Pediatric Orthopedics*, **18**, 304–311.

Davids, J.R., Holland, W.C., Sutherland, D.H. (1993) 'Significance of the confusion test in cerebral palsy.' *Journal of Peditric Orthopedics*, **3**, 717–721.

Dobson, F., Boyd, R.N., Parrott, J., Nattrass, G.R., Graham, H.K. (2002) 'Hip surveillance in children with cerebral palsy.' *Journal of Bone and Joint Surgery, British Volume*, **84**, 720–726.

Eliasziw, M., Young, S.L., Woodbury, M.G., Fryday-Field, K. (1994) 'Statistical methodology for the concurrent assessment of interrater and intrarater reliability: using goniometric measurements as an example.' *Physical Therapy*, **74**, 777–778.

Gage, J.R. (1992) *Gait Analysis in Cerebral Palsy. Clinics In Developmental Medicine No. 121.* London: Mac Keith Press.

Gentile, A.M. (1987) 'Skill acquisition: action, movement and neuromotor processes.' *In:* Carr, J.H., Shepherd, R.B., Gordon, J., Gentile, A.M., Held, J.M. (Eds.) *Movement Science: Foundations for Physical Therapy in Rehabilitation.* London: Heinemann Physiotherapy, pp. 93–154.

Hadders-Algra, M., Klip-Van Den Nieuwendijk, A.W.J., Martijn, A., Eykern, L.A. (1997) 'Assessment of general movements: towards a better understanding of a sensitive method to evaluate brain function in infants.' *Developmental Medicine and Child Neurology*, **39**, 89–99.

Haley, S.M., Coster, W.J., Faas, R.M. (1991) 'A content validity study of the Pediatric Evaluation of Disability Inventory.' *Pediatric Physical Therapy*, **3**, 177–184.

Kirschner, B., Guyatt, G. (1985) 'A methodological framework for assessing health indices.' *Journal of Chronic Disease*, **38**, 27–36.

Koman, L.A., Mooney, J.F., Smith, B.P., Goodman, A. (1994) 'Management of cerebral palsy with botulinum toxin A: report of a preliminary randomized, double blind trial.' *Journal of Pediatric Orthopedics*, **14**, 229–303.

Krunlinde-Sundholm, L., Eliasson, A-C. (2003) 'Development of the Assisting Hand Assessment: a Rasch built measure intended for children with unilateral upper limb impairments.' *Scandinavian Journal of Occupational Therapy*, **10**, 16–26.

Lacey, J.L., Henderson-Smart, D.J. (1998) 'Assessment of preterm infants in the intensive care unit to predict cerebral palsy and motor outcome at 6 years.' *Developmental Medicine and Child Neurology*, **40**, 310–318.

Landgraf, J.M., Abetz, L., Ware, J.A. (1996) *The CHQ User's Manual.* Boston: The Health Institute, New England Medical Centre.

Law, M., Baptiste, S., Cuswell, A., McColl, M., Polatajko, H., Pollack, M. (1994) *Canadian Occupational Performance Measure, 2nd Edn.* Toronto: Canadian Association of Occupational Therapy.

Law, M., King, G., Mackinnon, E, Russell, D., Murphy, C., Hurley, P., Bosch, E. (2001) *All About Outcomes: An Education Program to Help Understand, Evaluate and Choose Pediatric Outcome Measures (Individual). Version 1.0.* McMaster, Canada: Slack. (CD-ROM)

Love, S.C., Valentine, J.P., Blair, E.M., Price, C.J., Cole, J.H., Chauvel, P. (2001) 'The effect of botulinum toxin A on the functional ability of the child with spastic hemiplegia: a randomized controlled trial.' *European Journal of Neurology*, **8**, Suppl. 5, 178–182.

Mackie, A., Lobb, G., Walt, S., Stott, S. (2003) 'The reliability and validity of the Observational Gait Scale.' *Developmental Medicine and Child Neurology*, **45**, 4–11.

Maloney, F.P., Mirrett, P., Brooks, C., Johannes, K. (1978) 'Use of the Goal Attainment Scale in the treatment and ongoing evaluation of neurologically handicapped children.' *American Journal of Occupational Therapy*, **32**, 505–510.

McDowell, B.C., Hewitt, V., Nurse, A., Weston, T., Baker, R. (2000) 'The variability of goniometric measurements in ambulatory children with spastic cerebral palsy.' *Gait and Posture*, **12**, 114–121.

McLaughlin, J., Bjornsen, K., Temkin, N., Steinbok, P., Wright, V., Reiner, A., Roberts, T., Drakle, J., O'Donnell, M., Rosenbaum, P., Barber, J., Ferrel, A. (2002) 'Selective dorsal rhizotomy: meta-analysis of three randomized controlled trials.' *Developmental Medicine and Child Neurology*, **44**, 17–25.

McMulkin, M.L., Gulliford, J.J., Williamson, R.V., Ferguson, R.L. (2000) 'Correlation of static to dynamic measures of the lower extremity range of motion in cerebral palsy and control populations.' *Journal of Pediatric Orthopedics*, **20**, 366–369.

Novacheck, T. (2001) 'Management options for gait abnormalities.' *In:* Neville, B. (Ed.) *Congenital Hemiplegia. Clinics in Developmental Medicine No. 150*. London: Mac Keith Press, pp. 98–112.

Ounpuu, S., DeLucca, P.A., Davis, R.B. (2001) 'Gait analysis.' *In:* Neville, B. (Ed.) *Congenital Hemiplegia. Clinics in Developmental Medicine No. 150*. London: Mac Keith Press, pp. 81–97.

Parrott, J., Boyd, R.N., Dobson, F., Lancaster, A., Love, S., Oates, J., Wolfe, R., Nattrass, G.R., Graham, H.K. (2002) 'Hip displacement in spastic cerebral palsy: repeatability of radiological measurement.' *Journal of Pediatric Orthopedics*, **22**, 660–667.

Palisano, R., Rosenbaum, P., Walter, S., Russell, D., Wood E., Galuppi B (1997) 'Development and reliability of a system to classify gross motor function in children with cerebral palsy.' *Developmental Medicine and Child Neurology*, **39**, 214–223.

Perry, J. (1992) *Gait Analysis: Normal and Pathological Function*. Los Angeles: Slack.

Prechtl, H.F.R. (2001) 'General movement assessment as a method of developmental neurology: new paradigms and their consequences. The 1999 Ronnie Mac Keith Lecture.' *Developmental Medicine and Child Neurology*, **43**, 836–842.

Preston, C.C., Colman, A.M. (2000) 'Optimal number of response categories in rating scales: reliability, validity, discriminating power, and respondent preferences.' *Acta Psychologica*, **104**, 1–15.

Randall, M., Carlin, J.B., Chondros, P., Reddihough, D. (2001) 'Reliability of the Melbourne Assessment of Unilateral Upper-limb Function.' *Developmental Medicine and Child Neurology*, **43**, 761–767.

Rang, M. (1990) 'Cerebral palsy.' *In:* Morrissy, R.T. (Ed.) *Lovell and Winter's Pediatric Orthopedics, 3rd Edn*. Philadelphia: J.B. Lippincott, pp. 465–506.

Rodda, J., Graham, H.K. (2001) 'Classification of gait patterns in spastic hemiplegia and spastic diplegia: a basis for a management algorithm.' *European Journal of Neurology*, **8**, Suppl. 5, 98–108.

Rose, J., Gamble, J.G., Lee, J., Lee, R., Haskell, W.L. (1991) 'The Energy Expenditure Index: a method to quantitate and compare walking energy expenditure for children and adolescents.' *Journal of Pediatric Orthopaedics*, **11**, 571–578.

Rosenbaum, P.L., Walter, S.D., Hanna, S.E., Palisano, R.J., Russell, D.J., Raina, P., Wood, E., Bartlett, D.J., Galuppi, B.E (2002) 'Prognosis for gross motor function in cerebral palsy: creation of motor development curves.' *Journal of the American Medical Association*, **288**, 1357–1363.

Russell, D., Rosenbaum, P., Gowland, C., Hardy, S., Lane M., Plews N., McGavin H., Cadman, D., Jars, S. (1993) *The Gross Motor Function Measure, 2nd Edn*. Toronto: Hugh Macmillan Rehabilitation Center, McMaster University.

Russell, D.J., Avery, L.M., Rosenbaum, P.L. (2000) 'Improved scaling of the gross motor function measure for children with cerebral palsy: evidence of reliability and validity.' *Physical Therapy*, **80**, 873–885.

Ruwe, P.A., Gage, J.R., Ozonoff, M.B., DeLucca, P.A. (1992) 'Clinical determination of femoral anteversion.' *Journal of Bone and Joint Surgery, American Volume*, **74**, 820–830.

Sackett, D.L., Strauss, S.E., Rosenberg, W.S. (2001) *Evidence Based Practice: How to Practice and Teach EBM*. Edinburgh: Churchill Livingstone.

Sanger, T.D., Delgado M.R., Gaebler-Spira, D., Hallett, M., Mink, J.W. (2003) 'Classification and definition of disorders causing hypertonia in childhood.' *Pediatrics*, **111**, e89–97.

Scrutton, D., Baird, G. (1997) 'Surveillance measures of the hips in children with bilateral cerebral palsy.' *Archives of Disease in Childhood*, **56**, 381–384.

Scrutton, D., Baird, G.., Smeeton, N. (2001) 'Hip dysplasia in bilateral cerebral palsy: incidence and natural history in children aged 18 months to 5 years.' *Developmental Medicine and Child Neurology*, **43**, 586–600.

Stuberg, W.A., Fuchs, R.H., Meaner, J.A. (1988) 'Reliability of goniometric measurements of children with cerebral palsy.' *Developmental and Child Neurology*, **30**, 657–666.

Sutherland, D.H., Davids, J.R. (1993) 'Common gait abnormalities of the knee in cerebral palsy.' *Clinical Orthopaedics*, **288**, 139–147.

Sutherland, D.H., Olsen, R.A., Biden, E.N., Wyatt, M.P. (1988) *The Development of Mature Walking. Clinics in Developmental Medicine No. 104/105*. London: Mac Keith Press.

Tardieu, G., Shinto, S., Declare, R. (1954) 'A la recherché d'une technique de measure de la spasticité imprimé avec le periodique.' *Revue Neurologique*, **91**, 143–144.

WHO (2001) *International Classification of Impairments, Disabilities and Health.* Geneva: World Health Organization.

Wiley, M.E., Damiano, D.L. (1998) 'Lower-extremity strength profiles in spastic cerebral palsy.' *Developmental Medicine and Child Neurology*, **40**, 100–107.

Winters, T.F., Gage, J.R., Hicks, R. (1987) 'Gait patterns in spastic hemiplegia in children and young adults.' *Journal of Bone and Joint Surgery, American Volume*, **69**, 437–444.

6

NEURAL PLASTICITY AND LEARNING: THE POTENTIAL FOR CHANGE

Mary Galea

Development of sensorimotor systems and brain maps

Development is an ongoing, inexorable process, and has been likened to a ball rolling down a series of gullies (Waddington 1975). As development progresses, the environment in which it occurs also changes. At certain points the ball will take only one of several possible valleys and cannot reverse the process. This analogy, while useful, fails to take into account the importance of interaction in development. Interactions between cells, between groups of cells, and between the organism and the environment are critical factors in stimulating development. In the nervous system, neurons not only make synaptic contacts, but also interact with their targets, which may be other neurons or muscle fibres. This interaction appears to be critical for synapse formation. For example, at the neuromuscular junction, in addition to chemical signals operating in both directions between presynaptic and postsynaptic elements, neural (electrical) activity is important for the localization of acetylcholinesterase at the endplate (Lømo and Slater 1980). While the concept of functional specificity in the nervous system is important, *i.e.* particular neurons are always connected to particular targets, experience provides the major shaping stimulus in nervous system development (Edelman 1989). Connections between a neuron and its target are neither specified nor fixed. The precise connections of the nervous system depend on circumstances (Jacobsen 1991). Jean-Baptiste Lamarck (1744–1829) made plasticity, as a result of use and disuse, a central thesis of his theory of evolution: "The development of organs and their force or power of actions are always in direct relation to the employment of those organs" (cited in Jacobsen 1991).

PROLIFERATIVE AND REGRESSIVE PROCESSES IN NERVOUS SYSTEM DEVELOPMENT
After the initial proliferation of precursor cells and the sequence of divisions that give rise to neurons, the cells migrate from the site of origin to their final location where they undergo differentiation (extension of the axon and dendrites) and grow in size. Synapses begin to form around this time (for a review, see Shepherd 1994). Maturation of the neurons into their final form and function is a process that may take considerable periods of time. The development of neural connections in many regions of the central nervous system appears to be characterized by an initial overproduction of neurons, axons and synapses, followed at certain periods by the selective elimination or pruning of excess numbers of these structures (for a review, see Purves and Lichtman 1985).

Early in the prenatal period there is programmed neuronal cell death, where up to 50% of neurons initially formed will die (Oppenheim 1981). This process is a means of regulating cell numbers to match the capacity of the target structures, and corrects for some errors in positioning. Cells that survive appear to be successful in competing for growth factors. Thereafter neurons and their targets establish appropriate synaptic connections, avoiding potential synaptic partners that are in some sense incorrect. Normal behaviour requires precision in assembling these circuits, and it is not surprising that many disorders of behaviour are due to abnormalities in the development of appropriate connections. This selective synapse formation can be illustrated with reference to the connections of motor axons with different muscles and muscle fibre types (Schmidt and Stephani 1976) and the selective innervation of the homonymous spinal motoneurons by primary muscle afferents (Redman and Walmsley 1981). There appears to be a general principle that synaptic function precedes development of specialized synaptic structures. The immature cerebellar Purkinje cells of the rat respond to several putative neurotransmitters on days 1 and 2 after birth, yet synapses are not seen before day 3 postnatally (Woodward *et al.* 1971). Not all neurons in a given region differentiate, migrate and mature at the same time. In the cerebellar cortex, Purkinje cells take up their final positions long before the granule cells migrate and take on their final form. Failure of migration of the granule cells, as in the reeler mutant strain of mouse results in a lack of maturation of the characteristic dendritic tree of the Purkinje cells (Caviness and Rakic 1978). It appears that, in general, small interneurons arrive at their final location and mature after the projection neurons, and it has been suggested that small neurons and local synaptic circuits are more open to influence by experience (Shepherd 1994).

Dramatic increases in the connectivity of the mammalian cerebral cortex occur during the early postnatal period of development followed by synapse elimination. In the cerebral cortex of the macaque monkey, synaptic density increases during the last two prenatal months, reaches a peak about two months after birth and then decreases gradually to reach adult levels of synaptic density by about 3 years of age (Rakic *et al.* 1986). Synaptogenesis in the human visual cortex peaks at 2–4 months after birth and is followed by elimination of around 40% of synapses between the ages of 8 months and 11 years (Huttenlocher and De Courten 1987). What is lost in redundancy is gained in precision and efficiency.

NEURONAL SURVIVAL

Experiments involving investigation of muscle innervation or development of sensory systems have shown that the survival of neurons is dependent on functional synaptic contacts with their targets. There is a coincidence of neuronal cell death at the time at which the cells of that region are innervating their targets. In vertebrates this occurs because of competition between neurons at the level of the target they innervate. The competitive acquisition of trophic factors appears to be a common denominator of early neuron survival and later modulation of neuronal connections (Purves and Lichtman 1985). Removal of innervation leads to pronounced effects in the target neurons. An example is the response of the lateral geniculate nucleus (LGN) to visual deprivation. Removal of an eye or sewing the lid of one eye shut results in changes in the alternate layers of the LGN innervated alternately by inputs from the right and left eyes. In the affected layers, the size of the deprived neurons reduces markedly (Wiesel and Hubel 1963), and when this is done in young animals, some of these cells die (Kupfer and Palmer 1964). Another example is the neural pathway between the whiskers on the snouts of rats or mice and the cortical areas of representation of these receptors, the so-called 'barrel' fields. Each area in the barrel cortex responds to stimulation of a single whisker, even though three synaptic relays are interposed (Van der Loos and Woolsey 1973). Injury of a particular group of hair follicles at birth results in loss of the corresponding barrels in the cortex. Follicle injury at later ages appears to have little effect. These effects suggest that central neurons also depend on innervation for normal development.

SYNAPTIC REARRANGEMENT

Synaptic rearrangements in early life occur in many parts of the nervous system. These arrangements are designed to achieve the appropriate degree of convergence and divergence, and are also dependent on early experience (Shepherd 1994). Perhaps one of the most striking examples is the development of ocular dominance columns. In adult cats and monkeys, neurons in lamina IV of the primary visual cortex are segregated into columns dominated alternately by the right or left eye (Hubel *et al.* 1977). At birth there is considerable overlap of the geniculostriate terminals from each eye (Hubel *et al.* 1977), so that many of the neurons in lamina IV are driven by inputs from both eyes. The segregation of geniculostriate terminals into alternating bands occurs gradually by rearrangement of synapses and is dependent on visual experience. Occlusion of vision of one eye for the first three months leads to a change in the effectiveness of the occluded eye to drive visual cortical neurons. The geniculostriate terminals from this eye will contract, causing a reduction in visual abilities, while those from the normal eye will expand their territory. There are many other examples of similar processes occurring in the CNS. Projections across the corpus callosum are more diffuse in young animals and gradually become more restricted as a result of elimination of axon collaterals rather than by neuronal loss (O'Leary *et al.* 1981).

CRITICAL PERIODS

Although the patterns and strengths of synaptic connections in the nervous system are capable of some degree of relative adjustment throughout life, many connections pass through a period where the capacity for adjustment is substantially greater than in the adult brain. This period is referred to as a sensitive or critical period (Bateson 1979, Jacobsen 1991). A *sensitive period* is a developmental stage during which neurons select their permanent repertoire of inputs from a wider array of possible inputs. Experimentally, it is a period during which the anatomical and functional properties of neurons are particularly sensitive to modification by experience.

An extreme form of sensitive period is referred to as a *critical period*, a stage when appropriate experience is essential for the normal development of a pathway or set of connections. If appropriate experience is not gained during the critical period, the pathway never attains the ability to process information in a normal fashion, and therefore behaviour is permanently impaired (Jacobsen 1991). The developmental learning that occurs during critical periods can be distinguished from learning that occurs in adult animals in that the

69

changes occur readily only during a restricted period in the lifetime of an animal and persist throughout life. Greenough *et al.* (1993) suggest that this period is associated with 'experience-expectant' processes, *i.e.* the experiences obtained from the normal environment that shape developing sensory and motor systems of a species. This can be contrasted to 'experience-dependent' processes involving experiences that differ in both timing and character and that are unique to the individual. The neural manifestation of expectation or sensitivity appears to be the production of an excess number of synapses, a subset of which will be selectively preserved by experience-generated neural activity. If the normal pattern of experience occurs, a normal pattern of neural organization results. If an abnormal pattern of experience occurs, an abnormal pattern of neural organization will occur (Greenough *et al.* 1993).

DEVELOPMENT OF THE SENSORIMOTOR SYSTEM

The development of ocular dominance columns is an example of an activity-expectant process. Recent studies have highlighted a critical period for the development of motor systems, particularly of the corticospinal tract. Regressive events also characterize the development of the corticospinal projections. While the growth of axons towards their targets is completed in most systems by birth, the maturation of the corticospinal tract (CST) in mammals occurs largely postnatally. In the macaque monkey, there is a reduction in the population and areal extent of cortical neurons projecting to the spinal cord over the first few postnatal months (Galea and Darian-Smith 1995). Elimination of collateral projections rather than neuronal cell death is the likely mechanism for this reduction. At birth some axon terminals have already invaded the intermediate region but no other areas of the spinal grey matter. By 7–8 months, however, corticospinal axon terminals have their characteristic topography of termination in all regions of the spinal grey matter (Kuypers 1962, Galea and Darian-Smith 1995, Armand *et al.* 1997). Studies in the cat have shown that terminal and preterminal corticospinal axon branches increase in complexity during a protracted postnatal period, extending well beyond the period of refinement of the topography of terminations. Substantial branching and varicosity density have been identified before cortical motor circuits effectively drive their spinal targets (Li and Martin 2001)

Newborn primates, including man, have very poorly developed finger movements, and even basic hand skills take many months to acquire. These behavioural changes reflect, in part, the maturation of the neural substrate underlying control of the digits. While maturation of the structure of the corticospinal system coincides with the development of a precision grip between 3 and 6 months of age, a prolonged process of myelination means that adult values of conduction velocity are not attained until approximately 36 months (Olivier *et al.* 1997).

Neural activity in sensorimotor cortex has been found to be crucial in shaping postnatal development of corticospinal terminations in cats. Unilateral lesion of the corticospinal system during early postnatal life in cats and rats can result in aberrant corticospinal organization, with maintenance of exuberant projections from the non-damaged side (Hicks and D'Amato 1970, Leong and Lund 1973, Castro 1985, Leonard and Goldberger 1987b). Interference with neural activity in sensorimotor cortex by continuous infusion of muscimol, a $GABA_A$

agonist, in postnatal weeks 3–7 resulted in sparse corticospinal terminations to the contralateral spinal cord from the silenced area of cortex. Those from the active cortex maintained an immature bilateral pattern (Martin *et al*. 1999). Moreover, animals receiving unilateral muscimol infusions showed significant errors in reaching and grasping using the limb contralateral to the infusion. These behavioural deficits persisted despite further training and practice (Martin *et al*. 2000). Such infusions have also been found to affect limb loco-motor activity and postural reflexes (Leonard and Goldberger 1987a). These findings suggest that in the cat, the postnatal period between weeks 3 and 7 is a critical period for the maturation of corticospinal circuits for skilled motor control. Activity-dependent refinement of corticospinal axon terminations during this period is the mechanism whereby early motor experiences shape the structural and functional organization of the corticospinal system. Furthermore, the findings call to mind those of Hein (1974) in relation to kittens deprived of visual information about their limb movements. Such kittens failed to demon-strate normal visually guided behaviours in maturity. Martin *et al*. (2000) have suggested that prehension deficits resulting from sensorimotor cortex inactivation reflect a failure to integrate somatic sensory and perhaps visual information with the controlling elements driving the emerging movements, since the primary somatosensory cortex, particularly area 3a, the site of representation of afferent proprioceptive information, was also affected.

Cortical damage early in development in humans has also been shown to affect the functional organization of the corticospinal system. A different pattern of reorganization is observed if the perinatal lesions are unilateral rather than bilateral. Magnetic stimulation of the undamaged cortex following unilateral lesions produces bilateral motor responses, most probably through maintenance of ipsilateral corticospinal pathways (Benecke *et al*. 1991, Carr *et al*. 1993). It has been suggested that perinatal damage to one hemispheres disrupts the normal competition between contralateral and ipsilateral corticospinal projections, leading to abnormal preservation of the ipsilateral projections (Eyre *et al*. 2001). Such damage not only impairs the learning of motor skills but also secondarily disrupts the development of alpha motoneurons and their afferent segmental control (Myklebust *et al*. 1982, Leonard *et al*. 1991, Berger 1998, O'Sullivan *et al*. 1998). Activity in the early post-natal period affects the development of motoneuron soma size, dendritic morphology and pattern of synaptic inputs (Kalb and Hockfield 1992). Eyre *et al*. (2000) demonstrated that in humans, functional corticospinal connections are established prenatally, and may therefore play a role in the development of the spinal motoneurons.

All movements are essentially sensorimotor experiences, since movement generates sensory feedback, which, in turn, is instrumental in providing a constantly updated central representation of the body acting in the environment. Each corticospinal neuron population has a unique thalamic input that can relay particular sensorimotor information from the sense organs, cerebellum and basal ganglia. The overall structural framework of these sensorimotor pathways is that of many parallel corticospinal channels, with interconnections in the cere-bral cortex and spinal cord to enable cross-talk between channels. This is the basis for parallel distributed processing, which enables the very rapid transfer of information between the cerebral cortex and spinal cord needed for any sophisticated voluntary movement (Darian-Smith *et al*. 1996). Although thalamocortical projections to sensorimotor cortex are well established by birth, there is evidence for the pruning of exuberant terminal arborizations over the first few postnatal months (Darian-Smith *et al.* 1990). This process parallels that described earlier for the development of ocular dominance columns. Activity-dependent processes are also important in maintaining appropriate levels of activity in this pathway. Selective sensory deprivation induced by the trimming of two adjacent whiskers in neonatal rats results in abnormally low activity in the intracortical relay of inputs between lamina IV and the more superficial laminae II/III in barrel cortex (Rema *et al.* 2003).

When major modifications of sensory input occur early in life, massive changes in cortical organization can result. This is exemplified by observations of blind individuals in whom both braille reading (Sadato *et al.* 1996, Cohen *et al.* 1997, Büchel *et al.* 1998) and auditory localization tasks (Weeks *et al.* 2000) activate areas of cortex normally involved in visual processing. Similar types of cross-modal plasticity have been demonstrated in congenitally deaf individuals (Neville 1990). These findings imply that both natural and experimental modifications of peripheral influences early in life can result in a dramatic reassignment of sensory modalities to the cortical mantle within the life of an individual.

Theories of motor control and learning
Motor control models and theories have generally been developed around the issues of: (1) the basic units of nervous system organization relative to the basic units of motor function; and (2) principles applying to the organization of motor control.

REFLEX MODEL
The reflex model of motor control originated with Sherrington (1947) who found that specific stimuli such as stretch or pain induced distinct stereotyped movements called re-flexes (Fig. 6.1). An essential assumption of this model is that afferent input is a prerequisite for motor output. Later the concept of feedback in relation to motor control was introduced, with the notion that the human motor system might be controlled in ways similar to the control of mechanical systems. Servomechanisms are examples of systems that rely on feedback signals to maintain a stable output. Sherrington emphasized the importance of reflexes as elementary units of motor behaviour, with complex behaviour consisting of a successive combination or chaining of reflexes.

How are reflex pathways coordinated? Lundberg (1979) showed that different reflex pathways may share common interneurons. One of the best examples of this principle is the Ia interneuron, which not only mediates inhibition of antagonistic muscles in the stretch reflex, but is also part of an inhibitory pathway from flexor reflex afferents onto motoneurons. This neuron is a nodal point for control of spinal neurons by descending pathways (*e.g.* corticospinal, rubrospinal and vestibulospinal tracts) that are critical for skilled movement and postural control (Fig. 6.2) (Burke 1990).

HIERARCHICAL THEORY
The conceptual framework of a hierarchy has been of considerable influence in the analysis of motor control and for diagnosis in clinical neurology. The neurologist Hughlings Jackson (1835–1911) formulated the idea that there are successive levels of motor control in the

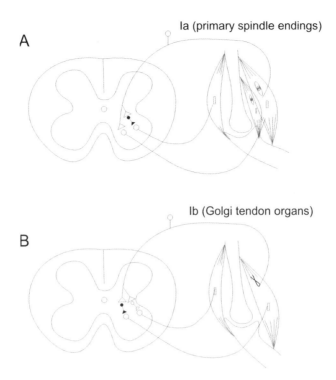

A

Ia (primary spindle endings)

B

Ib (Golgi tendon organs)

Fig. 6.1. Neural circuits for two types of spinal reflexes. Inhibitory terminals and interneurons are filled (black), while excitatory connections are unfilled (white).

A. Stretch reflex—detects phasic stretch of muscle and contributes to the control of movement.

B. Inverse myotatic reflex—detects tension and contributes to the control of muscle force and stiffness.

nervous system, with the control of automatic movements by lower levels and of purposive movements by higher levels. Higher levels normally exert control (either excitatory or inhibitory) over the lower levels. When higher level function is interrupted or destroyed by disease, the lower centres are 'released' from higher control. One of the consequences of this may be hyperactivity (such as exaggerated reflexes). It is now realized that motor control in the mammal is not strictly hierarchical. There are both *serial* and *parallel* pathways between regions of the nervous system, and motor control is *distributed*, that is, there are multiple representations of sensory and motor functions in the brain. The historical distinction between voluntary and reflex control is becoming increasingly blurred. For example, every voluntary movement is associated with automatic postural adjustments that occur unconsciously.

CLOSED-LOOP AND OPEN-LOOP SYSTEMS

Two basic systems have been described in the control of movement: feedback or closed-loop systems, and feedforward or open-loop systems (Schmidt 1982). Feedback control is usually

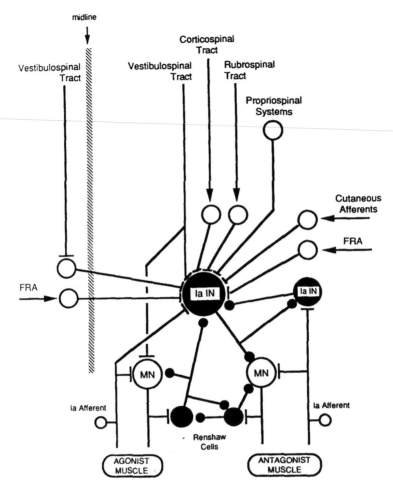

Fig. 6.2. Diagram illustrating the Ia inhibitory interneuron (Ia IN) as an integrating node in a number of spinal circuits. Excitatory neurons and synaptic terminals are indicated by open profiles, inhibitory by closed profiles.

FRA = flexor reflex afferents; MN = motoneuron; Ia afferent = sensory nerve from muscle spindle. (Adapted by permission from Burke 1990).

required for slow movements or those requiring accuracy. This type of control is characteristic of early skill acquisition. The linear view that underlies the idea of a closed-loop system (inputs, outputs, stimuli and responses, with feedback closing the loop) is only useful for simple systems. The concept of feedback in more complex systems is inadequate. Indeed, fluctuation between feedback and feedforward modes of control is typical of the control of movement in everyday life.

Feedforward control models involve the transfer of information to another part of the nervous system to 'prepare' it for impending motor commands. Examples of feedforward mechanisms are postural adjustments that precede self-initiated arm, leg and trunk movements to minimize any postural instability that would otherwise have resulted (Lee 1980, Frank and Earl 1990, Massion *et al*. 1982). This type of control is dependent on the nervous system having an accurate internal model of the body and the external environment. An inappropriate internal model can lead to poor predictions about the sensory consequences of situations and actions, resulting in anticipatory movements that are ineffective or cause loss of balance (Horak 1991).

MOTOR PROGRAMMES

The concept of a motor programme is based on an open-loop system of control and assumes that all movements are preplanned and stored in memory until required for action. Motor programmes have been defined as sets of muscle commands that are structured before a movement sequence begins, and that allow the entire movement sequence to be performed without the influence of peripheral feedback (Keele 1968). Studies of deafferentation in humans (Lashley 1917) and animals (Taub 1976) demonstrated that accurate movement was still possible in the absence of kinaesthetic information. One example of such programmes is the ability of the spinal cord to generate intrinsic rhythms or repeating patterns of muscle activity. Studies of both vertebrates and invertebrates have demonstrated that this property lies within neural circuits forming *central pattern generators*. Central pattern generators are recognized as key organizing principles for understanding rhythmical activities such as locomotion and respiration. These circuits generate essential rhythmical features of the motor pattern and receive sensory feedback signals.

SYSTEMS THEORY

If every individual neural and muscular component of the human body were controlled separately by the nervous system, this would be an enormous computational task. Bernstein (1967) introduced the concept of *degrees of freedom*. The more degrees of freedom in an activity, the more complicated the system and the more difficult it is to control. Thus, co-ordination in movement is the process of mastering redundant degrees of freedom* or making the system more controllable. Bernstein proposed that the nervous system does this by constraining groups of muscles to work together in synergies or coordinative structures. Examples of these synergies are the postural movement strategies, described by Horak and Nashner (1986), used to recover stability in response to brief displacements of the supporting surface (Fig. 6.3).

DYNAMICAL ACTION THEORY

The dynamical action theory, an elaboration of systems theory, proposes that movement *emerges* naturally out of the complex interactions among many interconnected elements (physical, environmental and neural), without specific commands or motor programmes in

*The number of dimensions in which a system can vary independently is known as the 'degrees of freedom'. The joints of the arm, excluding those of the hand, have seven degrees of freedom: the shoulder joint has three (flexion/extension, abduction/adduction, rotation), the elbow has two (flexion/extension, pronation/supination), and the wrist has two (flexion/extension, radial/ulnar deviation).

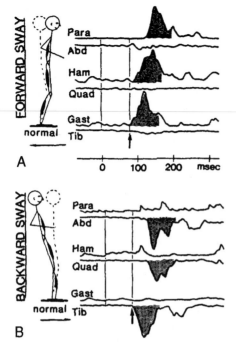

Fig. 6.3. Muscle synergy and body motion associated with the ankle strategy for controlling forward sway (A) and backward sway (B). (Reproduced by permission from Horak and Nashner 1986.)

the central nervous system. This theory brings the perspective of non-linear dynamics and synergetics to the question of how individual components such as neurons, muscles and joints of the body interact in such a way as to allow patterns of behaviour to emerge. These fields show in mathematically precise ways how complex systems may produce emergent order, that is, without a prescription for the pattern existing beforehand (Haken 1985), for example, in the formation of clouds, crystals and flow patterns in fluids.

At the core of the dynamical action theory is the notion that human behaviour is governed by a generic process of self-organization, which refers to the spontaneous formation of patterns and pattern change. The coordinative relations of various parts of a system, as well as the environment in which the interaction between the parts takes place are integral elements in this theory. The coordinative structures are the units of action, and are functionally linked, though not necessarily mechanically linked (Kelso and Tuller 1984). Using the framework of task dynamics, Saltzman and Kelso (1987) have suggested that the coordinative structures are constrained by the particular *tasks* that are being performed, and that the units of action are specified in *dynamic* terms rather than kinematic or muscular variables. Thus many features of an action, such as movement trajectory for example, are determined by the task. This theory differs from closed-loop models of control, which emphasize feedback, and from open-loop models of control, which emphasize the specifications for action; the dynamical perspective gives equal weight to both.

The dynamical perspective has important implications for the teaching of motor skills, and has also provided another view of motor development. Traditionally our understanding of how an infant acquires motor skills has been dominated by the idea of motor milestones, which are thought to reflect the infant's developing nervous system. This view emphasizes a deterministic sequence of behaviours mainly resulting from neural maturation, with the environment playing a minor role (Gesell 1945).

A dynamical systems approach, on the other hand, emphasizes the fact that many different subsystems contribute to the emerging motor behaviour. These systems include the infant's neurological, biomechanical and psychological maturation, but the behaviour also reflects the task being performed and its context. Since these systems mature at different rates, one or more of these may be so-called rate-limiting factors. Though many components contributing to a specific behaviour may be sufficiently developed, the behaviour may not emerge until the slowest component is sufficiently mature.

Thelen and colleagues (1987) have provided new insights into the development of human locomotion, showing that the process of learning to walk is both more complex and not as predictable as suggested by traditional views. They examined stepping behaviour in newborn infants, and noticed, contrary to the widely held belief that this behaviour disappeared in early infancy, that the same pattern continued in the kicking of infants lying on their back. Placing supported infants with their feet touching a treadmill elicited alternate stepping. At this stage, although the infants may possess the necessary neural connections and the ability to produce a specific movement pattern, they may have insufficient strength or postural control to demonstrate stepping under normal environmental conditions. However, when the infant is placed in water, where buoyancy removes the need to support body weight, the stepping patterns will re-emerge (Ulrich 1989). These step-like movements, of course, do not constitute walking, because walking requires the ability to support one's body against gravity. Following on from this, Heriza (1991) has proposed the following stages in the development of infant locomotion:
• pattern generation
• reciprocal flexor/extensor muscle activity
• anti-gravity strength in extensor muscles
• changes in body size and composition
• upright posture of head and trunk
• decoupling of early tight synchronization
• visual flow sensitivity while moving through the environment
• motivation towards a goal.

This list indicates a number of control parameters that govern transitions in behaviour in infancy. However, control parameters for developmental shifts may change at different ages and in different domains (Thelen 1993).

The coordination and control of action: learning and self-organization in the nervous system

The dynamical framework is useful in examining the issue of learning. The behaviour of complex systems such as a developing organism is dynamically stable in any given context, that is, behaviour fluctuates, but within limits (Fig. 6.4). Organisms tend to exhibit a certain number of behavioural patterns that will be the preferred states, and will be relatively re-

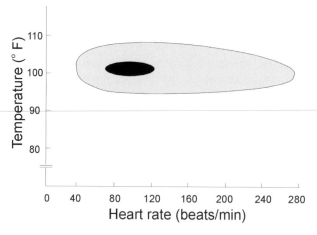

Fig. 6.4. A hypothetical representation of the dynamic range of heart rate and temperature. An individual will 'prefer' to spend time in the black centre portion, but is not limited to it. Perturbations, *e.g.* exercise or illness, may extend the heart rate and temperature into the grey region. (Adapted by permission from Thelen 1993.)

sistant to perturbation. In dynamic terminology, these are termed 'attractor' states. Using a non-biological example, a stretched spring will eventually stop at its equilibrium point. Complex systems may also switch between patterns in a discontinuous manner by exhibiting phase transitions. The onset of independent upright locomotion is an example of this. One day an infant cannot walk without support, and the next day he can toddle by himself.

The conceptual framework for modern approaches to the study of learning and memory is based on the notion that learning and memory must involve changes in neural circuits. Hebb (1949) postulated that learning and memory involve a change in synaptic efficacy between two neurons. This process might be relatively short-lived, or may persist and involve a structural change in the synapse, as in long-term potentiation or long-term depression, for example. The synapse is a complex functional unit, with a variety of time- and use-dependent controls. We have already seen that during development there is an enormous increase in the number of synapses, especially on the dendritic spines of cortical neurons. Cortical synapses are sensitive to environmental influences. Animals raised in enriched environments have thicker cortices and larger synaptic contacts, whereas environmental impoverishment leads to a reduction in the number of synapses and reduction in the size and complexity of individual synapses (Diamond *et al.* 1972). Context is therefore quite potent in promoting developmental change. For example, the ways that parents and caregivers relate and respond to young children, and the ways they mediate the infant's contact with the environment (*e.g.* providing access to objects, language opportunities etc.) will not only influence developing patterns of neuronal connectivity, but also provide a task context within which a child's developing subsystems may come together (Thelen 1993).

Learning theories have been predominantly concerned with two basic concepts as necessary conditions for learning: reinforcement (defined as some reward in the learning situation) and the nature of the sensory stimulus that causes the organism to respond. Traditionally, the theories have been classified as either associative (stimulus-response) or cognitive (Gestalt). Other motor learning theories postulate the development of a schema (Schmidt 1975) or a perceptual trace (Adams 1971) that is strengthened as a result of learning. The actual process of learning remains inaccessible to direct observation. Viewing learning as the mere strengthening of synaptic connections ignores the relationship between what is being learned and the intrinsic organization of the system that is learning. Sequential teaching of less complex patterns before more complex skills has been advocated, and is used in clinical practice (Larin 2000). However, reducing the difficulty of a task can alter the inherent nature of the skill to be learned. The framework of dynamical systems theory provides a view of learning that is quite different from this. Kelso (1995) has postulated that learning involves the emergence and stabilization of spatiotemporal patterns. Changes in behaviour with learning, traditionally measured in terms of improvement in performance of the task, are the outcome of modifications of the entire underlying dynamics (Kelso 1995)

Learning in the damaged nervous system

The review of sensorimotor development in the early postnatal period in the first section of this chapter shows that this is a period of enormous change. However there is increasing evidence that neural representations of body parts and movements are labile throughout life, changing according to the amount they are activated by peripheral inputs. This phenomenon has been most graphically demonstrated by the experiments of Merzenich and coworkers (1983, 1984), in which the reorganized cortical representations of the hand were mapped in the monkey following peripheral nerve lesions or digit amputation. These findings, and others illustrating similar reorganization in other cortical areas, indicate that topographic maps in the adult brain are not hard-wired, but can vary depending on spatial shifts in the collective activity of neurons with experience, a reorganization that is not haphazard but context dependent. The brain itself, therefore, can be viewed as a pattern-forming dynamical system (Kelso 1995).

The presence of a nervous system lesion or loss of appropriate stimulation at a critical period will lead to substantial alterations in the 'wiring' of the brain and altered behaviours. Children with cerebral palsy (CP) exhibit an immature non-plantigrade pattern of walking (Berger *et al*. 1982), the lack of heel strike resulting from premature activation of the calf muscles during the swing phase. In hemiplegic children these muscles produce just over a third of the positive work for the affected limb instead of the normal two thirds (Olney *et al*. 1990). The lack of push-off leads to the loss of the major propulsive force for the swing phase.

There are also impairments of upper-limb function in children with CP. Coupling of grip force and load force during lifting of an object does not develop in hemiplegic children. There is an early onset of excessive grip force and a lack of anticipatory control of the isometric force development during the load phase. It has been suggested that the early onset of and excessive grip force may compensate for the lack of anticipatory control and inefficient sensorimotor integration (Eliasson *et al*. 1991). The lack of anticipatory control may result from a poor internal representation of the object's physical properties due to disturbed sensory mechanisms (Gordon and Duff 1999).

These observations are consistent with the altered patterns of neural connections resulting from the brain lesion. Is learning possible in this situation? The dynamical systems theory provides a useful framework for examining motor skill acquisition in children with nervous system damage. Immature motor skills or actions have typically been viewed as representing a nervous system not yet able to carry out adaptive, coordinated movements. However, another perspective is to view immature motor actions as adaptive strategies to cope with immaturity in one or more of the contributing subsystems. Immature motor actions may also be the emergent consequences of biomechanical or other constraints that shape the movement (Bradley 1994). The notion of dynamic selection, proposed by Edelman (1989) has extended the dynamical action theory to incorporate three key elements. A developing organism has spontaneously generated behaviours that comprise the primary movement repertoire, and a sensory system capable of detecting and recognizing movements of adaptive value or importance. This will increase the probability of repetition of a movement ('selection') and therefore lead to changes in synaptic strength that will progressively modify the movement repertoire.

First, the environment must be examined to ensure that the developing system is receiving appropriate stimulation. Children with nervous system lesions will be more limited in their ability to explore the environment and to obtain appropriate sensorimotor experiences. Sensorimotor deprivation is likely to exacerbate the effects of nervous system lesions.

Second, possible constraints in certain subsystems that may limit motor behaviour should be explored. These constraints might be in the musculoskeletal system, as in the presence of spastic muscles (Dietz and Berger 1983), which are shorter and stiffer than normal muscles (Friden and Lieber 2003) and result in contractures. Abnormalities in the comparative rate of bone growth to muscle growth lead to muscle imbalances (Flett 2003) and subsequent biomechanical abnormalities (Rodda and Graham 2001). Weakness is one of the negative features of the upper motor neuron syndrome (Burke 1988) reflected in deficiencies in generating force and in sustaining force output (Bourbonnais and Vanden Noven 1989). Are these constraints amenable to manipulation? Contractures and their biomechanical sequelae have been managed with orthopaedic surgery. Following the removal of biomechanical constraints the child will have an opportunity for exploring new system relationships. It has been reported that it can take some children several months to regain mobility following single-event multi-level surgery (Morton 1999), indicating that change in one parameter may not be sufficient to effect a change in movement pattern. The presence of multiple constraints, including muscle weakness, is highly likely. Provision of strengthening exercises to children with CP has been shown to improve functional outcomes (Damiano and Abel 1998), supporting the view that muscle strength is an important control parameter for locomotion.

Third, the therapeutic and home environments must afford opportunities to practise tasks in a meaningful and functional context. The importance of context in the learning of motor skills is well known. Task-specific strengthening exercise and training for children with CP, run as a group circuit class, has been shown to result in improved strength and functional performance that is maintained over time (Blundell *et al.* 2003). During training, control parameters such as speed may be used to vary the task and facilitate exploration of a variety of movement patterns.

Learning to use the affected hand following unilateral cerebral lesions may present special difficulties. It has been reported that following such lesions in rats, neurons in the non-affected cortex became exceptionally responsive to changes in the behaviour of the non-affected forelimb. Such a response facilitated the learning of certain types of motor skills, and it was suggested that this behavioural compensation may contribute to the phenomenon of learned non-use of the impaired forelimb (Bury and Jones 2002).

Conclusion

Substantial changes take place in the central nervous system during infancy. Neuronal activity determines the morphological development of the nervous system. Appropriate sensorimotor experience is critical for the formation of cortical maps and for subsequent function. However, neural maturation alone is insufficient for development of motor function. A dynamical systems view emphasizes the fact that many different subsystems, neurological, musculoskeletal, perceptual, cognitive and emotional, contribute to emerging motor behaviour. Such a view provides a useful framework for examining the development of motor behaviour in children with central nervous system damage.

REFERENCES

Adams, J.A. (1971) 'A closed-loop theory of motor learning.' *Journal of Motor Behaviour*, **3**, 111–149.
Armand, J., Olivier, E., Edgely, S.A., Lemon, R.N. (1997) 'Postnatal development of corticospinal projections from motor cortex to the cervical enlargement in the macaque monkey.' *Journal of Neuroscience*, **17**, 251–266.
Bateson, P.P.G. (1979) 'How do sensitive periods arise and what are they for?' *Animal Behaviour*, **27**, 470–486.
Benecke, R., Meyer, B.U., Freund, H.J. (1991) 'Reorganisation of descending motor pathways in patients after hemispherectomy and severe hemispheric lesions demonstrated by magnetic brain stimulation.' *Experimental Brain Research*, **83**, 419–426.
Berger, W. (1998) 'Characteristics of locomotor control in children with cerebral palsy.' *Neuroscience and Biobehavioural Reviews*, **22**, 579–582.
Berger, W., Quintern, J., Dietz, J.V. (1982) 'Pathophysiology of gait in children with cerebral palsy.' *Electroencephalography and Clinical Neurophysiology*, **53**, 538–548.
Bernstein, N. (1967) *The Co-ordination and Regulation of Movements*. Elmsford, NY: Pergamon Press.
Blundell, S.W., Shepherd, R.B., Dean, C.M., Adams, R.D., Cahill, B.M. (2003) 'Functional strength training in cerebral palsy: a pilot study of a group circuit training class for children aged 4–8 years.' *Clinical Rehabilitation*, **17**, 48–57
Bourbonnais, D., Vanden Noven, S. (1989) 'Weakness in patients with hemiparesis.' *American Journal of Occupational Therapy*, **43**, 313–319.
Bradley, N.S. (1994) 'Motor control: developmental aspects of motor control in skill acquisition.' *In:* Campbell, S.K., Vander Linden, D., Palisano, R.J. (Eds.) *Physical Therapy for Children, 2nd Edn*. Philadelphia: W.B. Saunders, pp. 45–87.
Büchel, C., Price, C., Frackowiak, R.S., Friston, K. (1998) 'Different activation patterns in the visual cortex of late and congenitally blind subjects.' *Brain*, **121**, 409–419.
Burke, D. (1988) 'Spasticity as an adaptation to pyramidal tract injury.' *Advances in Neurology*, **47**, 401–423.
Burke, R.E. (1990) 'Spinal cord: ventral horn.' *In:* Shepherd, G.M. (Ed.) *The Synaptic Organization of the Brain*. New York: Plenum Press, pp. 88–132.
Bury, S.D., Jones, T.A. (2002) 'Unilateral sensorimotor cortex lesions in adult rats facilitate motor skill learning with the 'unaffected' forelimb and training-induced dendritic structural plasticity in the motor cortex.' *Journal of Neuroscience*, **22**, 8597–8606.

Carr, L.J., Harrison, L.M., Evans, A.L., Stephens, J.A. (1993) 'Patterns of central motor reorganization in hemiplegic cerebral palsy.' *Brain*, **116**, 1223–1247.

Castro, A.J. (1985) 'Ipsilateral corticospinal projections after large lesions of the cerebral hemisphere in neonatal rats.' *Experimental Neurology*, **46**, 1–8.

Caviness, V.S., Rakic, P. (1978) 'Mechanisms of cortical development: a view from mutations in mice.' *Annual Review of Neuroscience*, **1**, 297–326.

Cohen, L.G., Celnik, P., Pascual-Leone, A., Corwell, B., Falz, L., Dambrosia, J., Honda, M., Sadato, N., Gerloff, C., Catala, M.D., Hallett, M. (1997) 'Functional relevance of cross-modal plasticity in blind humans.' *Nature*, **389**, 180–183.

Damiano, D.l., Abel, M.F. (1998) 'Functional outcomes of strength training in children with cerebral palsy.' *Archives of Physical Medicine and Rehabilitation*, **79**, 119–125.

Darian-Smith, C., Darian-Smith, I., Cheema, S.S. (1990) 'Thalamic projections to sensorimotor cortex in the newborn macaque.' *Journal of Comparative Neurology*, **299**, 47–63.

Darian-Smith, I., Galea, M.P., Darian-Smith, C., Sugitani, M., Tan, A., Burman, K. (1996) 'The anatomy of manual dexterity. The new connectivity of the primate sensorimotor thalamus and cerebral cortex.' *Advances in Anatomy, Embryology and Cell Biology*, **133**.

Diamond, M.C., Rosenzwieg, M.R., Bennett, E.L., Lindner, B., Lyon, L. (1972) 'The effects of environmental enrichment and impoverishment on rat cerebral cortex.' *Journal of Neurobiology*, **3**, 47–64.

Dietz, V., Berger, W. (1983) 'Normal and impaired regulation of muscle stiffness in gait: a new hypothesis about muscle hypertonia.' *Experimental Neurology*, **79**, 680–687.

Edelman, G.M. (1989) *Neural Darwinism. The Theory of Neuronal Group Selection*. Oxford: Oxford University Press.

Eliasson, A.C., Gordon, A.M., Forssberg, H. (1991) 'Basic coordination of manipulative forces in children with cerebral palsy.' *Developmental Medicine and Child Neurology*, **33**, 659–668.

Eyre, J.A., Miller, S., Clowry, G.J., Conway, E.A., Watts, C. (2000) 'Functional corticospinal projections are established prenatally in the human foetus permitting involvement of spinal motor centres.' *Brain*, **123**, 51–64.

Eyre, J., Taylor, J., Villagra, F., Smith, M., Miller, S. (2001) 'Evidence of activity-dependent withdrawal of corticospinal projections during human development.' *Neurology*, **57**, 1543–1554.

Flett, P.J. (2003) 'Rehabilitation of spasticity and related problems in childhood cerebral palsy.' *Journal of Paediatric and Child Health*, **39**, 6–14.

Frank, J.S., Earl, M. (1990) 'Coordination of posture and movement.' *Physical Therapy*, **70**, 855–863.

Friden, J., Lieber, R.L. (2003) 'Spastic muscle cells are shorter and stiffer than normal cells.' *Muscle Nerve*, **27**, 157–164.

Galea, M.P., Darian-Smith, I. (1995) 'Postnatal changes in the direct corticospinal projections in the macaque monkey.' *Cerebral Cortex*, **5**, 518–540.

Gesell, A. (1945) *The Embryology of Behaviour*. New York: Harper. (Reprinted as *Classics in Developmental Medicine No. 3*, Mac Keith Press, London, 1988.)

Gordon, A.M., Duff, S.V. (1999) 'Fingertip forces during object manipulation in children with hemiplegic cerebral palsy. I: Anticipatory scaling.' *Developmental Medicine and Child Neurology*, **41**, 166–175.

Greenough, W.T., Black, J.E., Wallace, C.S. (1993) 'Experience and brain development.' *In:* Johnson, M.H. (Ed.) *Brain Development and Cognition. A Reader*. Oxford: Blackwell, pp. 290–319.

Haken, H. (1985) *Complex Systems: Operational Approaches in Neurobiology, Physics, and Computers*. Heidelberg: Springer.

Hebb, D.O. (1949) *The Organization of Behaviour*. New York: Wiley.

Hein, A. (1974) 'Prerequisite for development of visually-guided reaching in the kitten.' *Brain Research*, **71**, 259–263.

Heriza, C. (1991) 'Motor development: traditional and contemporary theories.' *In:* Lister, M.J. (Ed.) *Contemporary Management of Motor Control Problems. Proceedings of the II STEP Conference*. Alexandria, VA: Foundation for Physical Therapy, pp. 99–126.

Hicks, S.P., D'Amato, C.J. (1970) 'Motor-sensory and visual behaviour after hemispherectomy in newborn and mature rats.' *Experimental Neurology*, **29**, 416–438.

Horak, F. (1991) 'Assumptions underlying motor control for neurologic rehabilitation.' *In:* Lister, M.J. (Ed.) *Contemporary Management of Motor Control Problems. Proceedings of the II Step Conference*. Alexandria, VA: Foundation for Physical Therapy, pp. 11–27.

Horak, F., Nashner, L. (1986) 'Central programming of postural movements: adaptation to altered support surface configurations.' *Journal of Neurophysiology*, **55**, 1369–1381.

Hubel, D.H., Wiesel, T.N., LeVay, S. (1977) 'Plasticity of ocular dominance columns in the monkey striate cortex.' *Philosophical Transactions of the Royal Society of London. Series B: Biological Sciences*, **278**, 377–409.

Huttenlocher, P.R., De Courten, C. (1987) 'The development of synapses in striate cortex of man.' *Human Neurobiology*, **6**, 1–9.

Jacobsen, M. (1991) *Developmental Neurobiology, 3rd Edn.* New York: Plenum Press.

Kalb, R.G., Hockfield, S. (1992) 'Activity-dependent development of spinal cord motor neurons.' *Brain Research. Brain Research Reviews*, **17**, 283–289.

Keele, S.W. (1968) 'Movement control in skilled motor performance.' *Psychological Bulletin*, **70**, 387–403.

Kelso, J.A.S. (1995) *Dynamic Patterns. The Self-Organization of Brain and Behaviour.* Cambridge, MA: MIT Press.

Kelso, J.A.S., Tuller, B. (1984) 'A dynamical basis for action systems.' *In:* Gazzaniga, M. (Ed.) *Handbook of Cognitive Neuroscience.* New York: Plenum Press, pp. 321–356.

Kupfer, C., Palmer, P. (1964) 'Lateral geniculate nucleus: histological and cytochemical changes following afferent denervation and visual deprivation.' *Experimental Neurology*, **9**, 400–409.

Kuypers, H.G.J.M. (1962) 'Corticospinal connections: Postnatal development in the rhesus monkey.' *Science*, **138**, 678–680.

Larin, H. (2000) 'Motor learning theories and strategies for the practitioner.' *In:* Campbell, S.K., Vander Linden, D., Palisano, R.J. (Eds.) *Physical Therapy for Children, 2nd Edn.* Philadelphia: W.B. Saunders, pp. 170–197.

Lashley, K.S. (1917) 'The accuracy of movement in the absence of excitation from the moving organ.' *American Journal of Physiology*, **43**, 169–194.

Lee, W. (1980) 'Anticipatory control of postural and task muscles during rapid arm flexion.' *Journal of Motor Behaviour*, **12**, 185–196.

Leonard, C.T., Goldberger, M.E. (1987a) 'Consequences of damage to sensorimotor cortex in neonatal and adult cats. I. Sparing and recovery of function.' *Brain Research. Developmental Brain Research*, **32**, 1–14.

Leonard, C.T., Goldberger, M.E. (1987b) 'Consequences of damage to sensorimotor cortex in neonatal and adult cats. II. Maintenance of exuberant projections.' *Brain Research. Developmental Brain Research*, **32**, 15–30.

Leonard, C.T., Hirschfeld, H., Moritani, T., Forssberg, H. (1991) 'Myotatic reflex development in normal children and children with cerebral palsy.' *Experimental Neurology*, **111**, 379–382.

Leong, S.K., Lund, R. (1973) 'Anomalous bilateral corticofugal pathways in albino rats after neonatal lesions.' *Brain Research*, **62**, 218–221.

Li, Q., Martin, J.H. (2001) 'Postnatal development of corticospinal axon terminal morphology in the cat.' *Journal of Comparative Neurology*, **435**, 127–141.

Lømo, T., Slater, C.R. (1980) 'Control of junctional acetylcholinesterase by neural and muscular influences in the rat.' *Journal of Physiology*, **303**, 191–202.

Lundberg, A. (1979) 'Integration in a propriospinal motor centre controlling the forelimb in the cat.' *In:* Asanuma, H., Wilson, V.J. (Eds.) *Integration in the Nervous System.* Tokyo: Igaku-Shoin, pp. 47–64.

Martin, J.H., Kably, B., Hacking, A. (1999) 'Activity-dependent development of cortical axon terminations in the spinal cord and brain stem.' *Experimental Brain Research*, **125**, 184–199.

Martin, J.H., Donarummo, L., Hacking, A. (2000) 'Impairments in prehension produced by early postnatal sensory motor cortex activity blockade.' *Journal of Neurophysiology*, **83**, 895–906.

Massion, J., Hugon, M., Wiesendanger, M. (1982) 'Anticipatory postural changes induced by active unloading and comparison with passive unloading in man.' *Pflügers Archives*, **393**, 292–296.

Merzenich, M.M., Kaas, J.H., Wall, J.T., Nelson, R.J., Sur, M., Felleman, D.J. (1983) 'Topographic reorganization of somatosensory cortical areas 3b and 1 in adult monkeys following restricted deafferentation.' *Neuroscience*, **8**, 33–55.

Merzenich, M.M., Nelson, R.J., Stryker, M.P., Cynader, M.S., Shoppmann, A., Zook, J.M. (1984) 'Somatosensory cortical map changes following digit amputation in adult monkeys.' *Journal of Comparative Neurology*, **224**, 591–605.

Morton, R. (1999) 'New surgical interventions for cerebral palsy and the place for gait analysis.' *Developmental Medicine and Child Neurology*, **41**, 424–428.

Myklebust, B.M., Gottlieb, G.L., Penn, R.D., Agarwal, G.C. (1982) 'Reciprocal excitation of antagonistic muscles as a differentiating feature in spasticity.' *Annals of Neurology*, **12**, 367–374.

Neville, H.J. (1990) 'Intermodal competition and compensation in development. Evidence from studies of the visual system in congenitally deaf adults.' *Annals of the New York Academy of Sciences*, **608**, 71–87.

O'Leary, D.D.M., Stanfield, B.B., Cowan, W.M. (1981) 'Evidence that early postnatal restriction of the cells of origin of the callosal projection is due to the elimination of axonal collaterals rather than to the death of neurons.' *Developmental Brain Research*, **1**, 607–617.

Olivier, E., Edgely, S.A., Armand, J., Lemon, R.N. (1997) 'An electrophysiological study of the postnatal development of the corticospinal system in the macaque monkey.' *Journal of Neuroscience*, **17**, 267–276.

Olney, S.J., MacPhail, H.E., Hedden, D.M., Boyce, W.F. (1990) 'Work and power in hemiplegic cerebral palsy gait.' *Physical Therapy*, **70**, 431–438.

Oppenheim, R.W. (1981) 'Neuronal cell death and some related regressive phenomena during neurogenesis: A selective historical review and a progress report.' *In:* Cowan, W.M. (Ed.) *Studies in Developmental Neurobiology. Essays in Honor of Viktor Hamburger*. New York: Oxford University Press, pp. 74–133.

O'Sullivan, M.C., Miller, S., Ramesh, V., Conway, E., Gilfillian, K., McDonough, S., Eyre, J.A. (1998) 'Abnormal development of biceps brachii phasic stretch reflex and persistence of short latency heteronymous reflexes from biceps to triceps brachii in spastic cerebral palsy.' *Brain*, **121**, 2381–2395.

Purves, D., Lichtman, J.W. (1985) Principles of Neural Development. Sunderland, MA: Sinauer Associates.

Rakic, P., Bourgeois, J-P., Eckenhoff, M.F., Zecevic, N., Goldman-Rakic, P. (1986) 'Concurrent overproduction of synapses in diverse regions of the primate cerebral cortex.' *Science*, **232**, 232–235.

Redman, S., Walmsley, B. (1981) 'The synaptic basis of the monosynaptic stretch reflex.' *Trends in Neurosciences*, **4**, 248–251.

Rema, V., Armstrong-James, M., Ebner, F.F. (2003) 'Experience-dependent plasticity is impaired in adult rat barrel cortex after whiskers are unused in early postnatal life.' *Journal of Neuroscience*, **23**, 358–366.

Rodda, J., Graham, H.K. (2001) 'Classification of gait patterns in spastic hemiplegia and spastic diplegia: a basis for a management algorithm.' *European Journal of Neurology*, Suppl. 5, 98–108.

Sadato, N., Pascual-Leone, A., Grafman, J., Ibanez, V., Deiber, M.P., Dold, G., Hallett, M. (1996) 'Activation of the primary visual cortex by Braille reading in blind subjects.' *Nature*, **380**, 526–528.

Saltzman, E., Kelso, J.A.S. (1987) 'Skilled actions: a task-dynamic approach.' *Psychological Review*, **94**, 84–106.

Schmidt, H., Stephani, E. (1976) 'Re-innervation of twitch and slow muscle fibres of the frog after crushing the motor nerves.' *Journal of Physiology*, **270**, 507–517.

Schmidt, R.A. (1975) 'A schema theory of discrete motor skill learning.' *Psychological Review*, **82**, 225–260.

Schmidt, R.A. (1982) *Motor Control and Learning. A Behavioural Emphasis*. Champaign, IL: Human Kinetics.

Shepherd, G.M. (1994) *Neurobiology, 3rd Edn*. New York: Oxford University Press.

Sherrington, C.S. (1947) *The Integrative Action of the Nervous System, 2nd Edn*. Cambridge: Cambridge University Press.

Taub, E. (1976) 'Movements in non-human primates deprived of somatosensory feedback.' *Exercise and Sports Science Reviews*, **4**, 335–374.

Thelen, E. (1993) 'Self-organization in developmental processes: can systems approaches work?' *In:* Johnson, M.H. (Ed.) *Brain Development and Cognition. A Reader*. Cambridge, MA: Blackwell, pp. 555–591.

Thelen, E., Kelso, J.A.S., Fogel, A. (1987) 'Self-organizing motor systems and infant motor development.' *Developmental Review*, **7**, 39–65.

Ulrich, B. (1989) 'Development of stepping patterns in human infants: a dynamical perspective.' *Journal of Motor Behaviour*, **21**, 392–408.

Van der Loos, H., Woolsey, T.A. (1973) 'Somatosensory cortex: structural alterations following early injury to sense organs.' *Science*, **179**, 395–398.

Waddington, C.H. (1975) *The Evolution of an Evolutionist*. Edinburgh: Edinburgh University Press.

Weeks, R., Horwitz, B., Aziz-Sultan, A., Tian, B., Wessinger, C.M., Cohen, L.G., Hallett, M., Rauschecker, J.P. (2000) 'A positron emission tomographic study of auditory localization in the congenitally blind.' *Journal of Neuroscience*, **20**, 2664–2672.

Wiesel, T.N., Hubel, D.H. (1963) 'Effects of visual deprivation on morphology and physiology of cells in the cat's lateral geniculate body.' *Journal of Neurophysiology*, **26**, 978–993.

Woodward, D.J., Hoffer, B.J., Siggins, G.R., Bloom, F.E. (1971) 'The ontogenetic development of synaptic junctions, synaptic activation and responsiveness to neurotransmitter substances in rat cerebellar Purkinje cells.' *Brain Research*, **34**, 73–97.

7
THE ASSESSMENT AND MANAGEMENT OF HYPERTONUS IN CEREBRAL PALSY: A PHYSIOLOGICAL ATLAS ('ROAD MAP')

Jean-Pierre Lin

For over a hundred years, there has been a keen clinical interest in altering muscle tone in an attempt to bring about functional gains in cerebral palsy (CP). Over this period, the natural history of CP has changed considerably with a marked reduction in postnatally acquired forms attributable to childhood infections which would have provided the bulk of William Osler's case series (Osler 1889). Most cases of CP now find their origins pre-natally (Stanley *et al*. 2000). Despite these prenatal origins, the majority of children with CP are born at term and the dominant cerebral insult is bilateral periventricular leukomalacia (PVL) (for a general review of the cerebral palsies, see Lin 2003). The classification of the cerebral palsies has been largely clinical (Mutch *et al*. 1992), with recourse to occasional post-mortem studies (Freud 1897, Christensen and Melchior 1967). A more up-to-date review of the neuropathology in relation to timing of injury can be found in Waney Squier's excellent book (2002). Imaging studies (for reviews, see Krageloh-Mann 2000, Anslow 2002, Rutherford 2002) will increasingly contribute to a coherent strategy, linking together with the timing of injury, neuropathology, neurophysiology and clinical symptomatology, for success in clinical management.

Operational definitions
Clinically, 'muscle tone' is described as the resistance felt when a limb is passively rotated about a joint with the subject at rest. Most clinicians will recognize that 'muscle tone' is affected both by the state of arousal of the subject and by the context or conditions under which it is assessed. In addition, the clinical definition of 'hypertonus' is very much user-dependent. Most of us also recognize that what matters most is the possible interference of abnormal postures and tone with voluntary movements, rather than the passive stretching of muscles during a couch assessment. Hence, this chapter concentrates on building up a *physiological atlas* of the different components of 'muscle tone', each of which has a sep-arate operational definition that allows the observer to detect and quantify an event or process and to record it reliably. The purpose of this atlas is to focus on different physiological problems and their potential solutions.

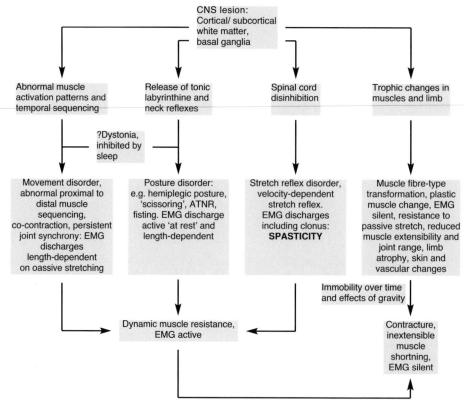

Fig. 7.1. Clinical assessment of motor function and muscle tone. The contribution of muscle sequencing patterns, abnormal postures, reflex excitability and intramuscular changes is shown. Trophic changes in muscle and limb are very much an 'end-stage' or the culmination of a combination of disuse during periods of active bone growth. The aim of all management is to promote movement and strength while preventing immobility, disuse and deformity. In practice these clinical phenomena coexist to varying degrees in most children and adults with CP. (Reproduced by permission from Lin 2000.)

The motor syndrome of cerebral palsy

Children with CP experience varying degrees of limitation in their motor skills. Disordered motor performance may be divided into the following categories according to an anatomical and physiological hierarchy in descending order from 'brain to bone':

1. Delayed motor development and weakness
2. Impaired movement sequencing, dexterity, anticipatory control
3. Inappropriate postures and associated postures
4. Exaggerated reflex excitability and spasms
5. Muscular biomechanical transformation: changes in visco-elastic properties
6. Bone and joint deformity as the child grows.

   Figure 7.1 summarizes the mechanisms of motor impairment according to a physiological scheme. These phenomena should be seen as coexisting rather than in isolation from each other. For instance, inappropriate postures are likely to result in poor motor performance on the one hand, and may produce fixed deformity (contracture) on the other. Once deformity becomes fixed, further deterioration in posture and function follow. For many clinicians, all of these variables are reduced to a single term such as 'spastic syndrome' or 'dystonia', but it will be argued here that children with CP have an evolving disorder of movement and posture of which the disordered 'tone' is but one component.

WEAKNESS AND POOR SELECTIVE MOTOR CONTROL
Muscle strength depends on a combination of central and peripheral interactions. A detailed discussion of the underlying mechanisms is beyond the scope of this chapter (see Chapter 11 for further details on muscle strengthening) but the firing properties of the first-order motorneuron, the large Betz cells in the precentral gyrus of the contralateral hemisphere and their connections to the lower motorneuron are essential to generating muscle force. Put simply, a depleted population of Betz cells, or reduced connections because of white matter wasting, or alterations in the firing frequencies of the cells, results in a reduced force output (see Evarts 1968). Figure 7.2 shows the effect of weakness in quiet standing, with abolition of EMG output during swaying.

There are interesting relationships between voluntary control, limb length, inertia, and adaptations to growth and muscle stiffness or damping. If the system is over-damped (increased muscle stiffness), the range of movement will be limited. If under-damped, excessive or wild movements may ensue. Limbs that perform smooth cyclical movements tend to have high inertia and low muscle stiffness. Limbs designed to perform fine, non-repetitive and complex movements tend to have low inertia and high muscle stiffness. Toddlers produce inaccurate movements for a variety of reasons, including immature motor patterns and high muscle compliance. Under-damped limbs, characterized by excessive compliance, contribute to poor motor control. In addition to increased muscle compliance, the limbs of toddlers and young children have very little inertia (see Table 7.3, p. 96). Inertial damping stabilizes movements and helps to reduce unwanted oscillations. Motor performance is often greatly impaired in the presence of low limb inertia and hypotonia.

ABNORMAL MOTOR SEQUENCES, WITH PARTICULAR REFERENCE TO CO-CONTRACTION
Co-contraction may be developmental, physiological or pathological, or all three combined.

Developmental co-contraction that may persist in CP
Both for voluntary muscle function and in response to sudden perturbations, the healthy motor system produces consistently observable patterns that are disturbed with damage to the CNS. A dominant motor pattern is that of co-contraction of agonist and antagonist muscle groups. Observations of the developing healthy infant show that co-contraction is the norm in the first two years of life. Such co-contraction benefits the development of postural stability at the expense of mobility. Excessive limb flexion as seen in a physiological crouch stance or crouch gait also offers additional postural stability but cannot be sustained for other than short periods, which is why young toddlers stand and walk for brief periods before

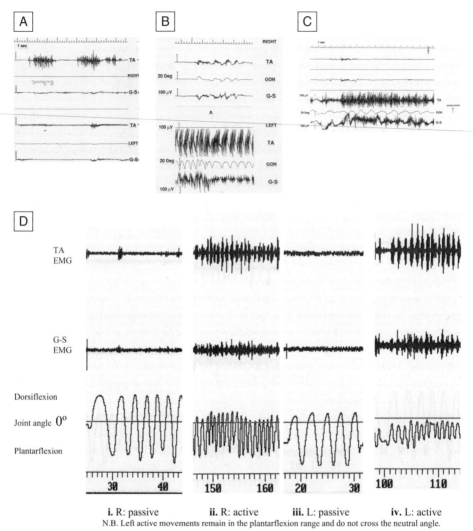

i. R: passive   **ii.** R: active   **iii.** L: passive   **iv.** L: active
N.B. Left active movements remain in the plantarflexion range and do not cross the neutral angle.

Fig. 7.2. Weakness, poverty of motor output and reduced fine motor dexterity.

    A. *Weakness in standing: the good leg does all the work.* The right (unaffected) leg shows bursts of EMG in the tibialis anterior as this 12-year-old girl with left hemiplegia sways gently on her legs. The left hemiparetic leg is relatively unresponsive during weight bearing.

    B. *Weakness of right leg during voluntary alternating movements at the ankle.* Voluntary alternating ankle movements in a 10-year-old girl with right hemiplegia. Attempted movements on the right (upper traces) produce a feeble EMG output of low amplitude, slowly firing motor units that produce low muscle force and hence poorly differentiated movements of low amplitude in contrast to the vigorous movements at the left ankle (lower traces).

    C. 12-year-old girl with left hemidystonia. This dystonic leg has great difficulty producing alternating movements at the ankle: in this case the EMG output is overwhelming and discrete movements are impossible.

Continued opposite ↗

88

returning to the safety of the ground. Movements are necessarily brief, jerky and stiff, and characterized by joint synchronies. With the development of unsupported walking, co-contraction diminishes, movements become more graceful, and functional joint asynchronies emerge. If a child has a non-progressive lesion to the developing brain (CP), muscle co-contraction or co-activation persists into the unsupported walking phase (Leonard *et al.* 1991), *i.e. mobility is sacrificed in favour of stability.*

Additional light is shed on the maturation of muscle activation patterns by the work of Sutherland *et al.* (1988) who demonstrated that among healthy children, two-thirds of 1-year-olds and one-third of 7-year-olds exhibited prolonged muscle activation patterns during the gait cycle. The gastrocnemius muscle, for instance, was inappropriately active in the swing phase of gait, thus producing plantarflexion in terminal swing at a time when dorsiflexion is required preparatory to heel contact. There is therefore a powerful developmental context for co-contraction and prolonged muscle activation, which persists in some people for prolonged periods of childhood. An additional physiological explanation for co-contraction of muscles lies in the observation that passive muscle compliance is extremely high among toddlers and diminishes with age (Lin *et al.* 1997) (Fig. 7.3). Thus, the muscles of infants and toddlers are if anything excessively compliant, requiring co-contraction to increase joint stability. Our muscles stiffen up over the first decade. Co-contraction may be essential to make up for the lack of 'passive tone'. The motor performance of children with hypotonia and/or joint laxity is notoriously poor and slow to develop, and the quality of achieved movements is poor. This may be because of the need to harness excessive co-contraction to the task because of a lack of the appropriate passive muscle tone (reduced rheological resistance). In addition, the twitch times of muscles of young children are ex-

---

D. *Alternating voluntary plantarflexion–dorsiflexion movements at the ankle: frequency and amplitude restricted by muscle stiffness and contracture.* Traces from an 8-year-old girl with congenital left hemiplegia.
  i. Passive alternating movements at the right ankle: the foot can be dorsiflexed well beyond 0° (when the foot is at right angles to the shank).
 ii. Normal voluntary alternating movements at the right ankle: note that these rapid movements include dorsiflexion beyond neutral. In fact, for healthy subjects the angular motion has large amplitude at slow frequencies and small amplitude at fast frequencies because angular acceleration is proportional to the square of the frequency and the amplitude of motion is inversely proportional to the square of the frequency of movements. Of particular note is that the fastest movements occur about the neutral axis, *i.e.* when the ankle is neither plantarflexed nor dorsiflexed. This is accompanied by recruitment of the largest and fastest firing motor units (see Lin *et al.* 1996a).
iii. Passive alternating movements at the left ankle: the foot can just be dorsiflexed beyond the 0° angle, *i.e.* passive movements are restricted on the hemiparetic side.
  Voluntary alternating movements of the hemiparetic ankle are restricted in amplitude, do not cross the 0° angle into anatomical dorsiflexion and are of lower frequency than on the healthy right side. This hemiparetic leg does not have the poverty of EMG output shown in (B). Some of this 'weakness' is attributable to intrinsic muscle stiffness and a restricted joint range. The resonant frequency at the ankle of the hemiparetic leg was 4 Hz compared with 3.4 Hz at the healthy ankle (see Table 7.3 for details about resonant frequency).
  G-S EMG = gastrocnemius–soleus muscle surface EMG.
  TA EMG = tibialis anterior muscle surface EMG.

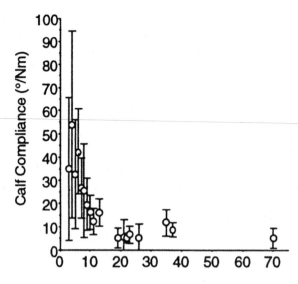

Fig. 7.3. Reduction in muscle compliance with age in healthy subjects. Joint compliance reduces with age, *i.e.* quiescent muscles get stiffer as children get older. The excessive muscle compliance (reduced passive tone) is associated with poor motor performance and excessive co-contraction of agonist–anatagonist muscle pairs. (Reproduced by permission from Lin *et al*. 1997.)

ceptionally prolonged (Lin *et al*. 1994b), providing further compensation to excessive compliance.

In addressing the issue of how to manage hypertonus, it is essential to assess whether it is developmentally appropriate for function. Developmental co-contraction in children with CP is bound to be detected in gait laboratories and may result in decisions for intervention. Clinicians should ask the questions: "What is the functional significance of co-contraction (muscle tone) in this child?" and "Does this co-contraction support or impede function?"

Walking speed, prolonged muscle activation and co-contraction
As walking speed increases, so the EMG activation of a number of leg muscles is prolonged (Detrembleur *et al*. 1997). This necessarily alters the stiffness of the limbs during the gait cycle, dynamic stiffness increasing with increasing speed of walking. Children with CP are said to walk as if in a hurry. If the walking EMG patterns are collected while employing these self-selected hasty walks, increasing co-contraction with increasing velocity of gait will be observed. Comparisons of walking before and after intervention should attempt to control for walking speed. In this instance, training to walk more slowly may reduce co-contraction stiffness.

Muscle activation patterns in response to perturbations of posture
Children with bilateral CP are often described as prone to falling. 'Poor balance', 'muscle

stiffness' and an 'inadequate base of support' are phrases often used to explain their instability. A remarkable physiological pattern of muscle activation was discovered by Nashner *et al.* (1983) in studies using tilt platforms. He showed that healthy children always stabilize the ankle joint first followed by the knee joint later. In other words, a strategy of 'distal-to-proximal' muscle activation patterns is generated that has the effect of stabilizing the segment of the limb closest to the tilting platform. This distal-to-proximal pattern of muscle activation obtained whether the subject was tilted forwards, when gastrocnemius activation preceded hamstring muscle activation, or tilted backwards, when tibialis anterior activation preceded quadriceps muscle activation.

By contrast, children with hemiplegia or diplegia demonstrated a 'proximal-to-distal' sequencing pattern of muscle activation when the subjects were tilted forwards or backwards, *i.e.* thigh muscle activation always preceded below-knee muscle activation, leaving the distal segment (ankle joint) effectively flail for a fraction of time sufficient to allow the subject to be unstable. No abnormalities in the muscle activation patterns were found in the uninvolved leg of hemiplegic children or in either leg of the ataxic children, even though ataxic children did produce the greatest sway on being perturbed. This pattern has nothing to do with 'spasticity' or 'dystonia' but illustrates an inappropriate central efferent command in response to perturbation. Nashner (1985) concluded: "The results of moving platform assessment support the contention that pathological changes in stretch reflex mechanisms associated with spasticity are secondary to the primary functional loss: namely, alterations in central and spinal programs which impose the appropriate temporal and spatial structures upon motor activities of the limb prior to the execution of the task."

DISORDERED POSTURES

Postures are centrally driven, often complex, sustained limb attitudes that vary according to severity of the motor disorder and motor development. They are also task-dependent and may alter according to specific and nonspecific afferent input as well as the state of arousal. A simple classification of posture is listed:

A. Embryological and developmental considerations: postural stages of man

The developing human fetus goes through several obligate opposing extensor and flexor postural stages over the first 40 weeks of development (Brown *et al.* 1997). These are lost with cerebral maturation but may return with CNS damage, *e.g.* paraplegia in flexion or extension.

B. Associated postures

There are a number of postures accompanying tasks or generated by certain positions in relation to the action of gravity, either indirectly through the vestibular apparatus or directly on weak muscles.

i. Compensatory postures associated with balancing: use of inertia management strategies

These postures are aimed at increasing stability at the expense of unwanted mobility, by reducing the available degrees of freedom of movement, and will be produced by upper and lower limb co-contraction strategies.

ii. Føg posturing: associated with motor maturation

Some children (*e.g.* most 4-year-olds and up to 25% of 16-year-olds) will adopt involuntary associated postures of their arms and hands when asked to perform unfamiliar walks (Føg and Føg 1963). 'Føg postures' are usually signs of motor immaturity in the developing child, are exaggerated in children with learning difficulties and in children with motor impairments.

iii. Posture and the influence of tonic labyrinthine and tonic neck inputs

Cortical strokes produce gravity-assisted wrist postures with the wrist pronated. The arm is adducted and internally rotated at the shoulder, and flexed at the elbow and metacarpophalangeal joints. This is not simply due to weakness, but also due to 'tonic' supraspinal and cervical influences increasing the continuous activity of certain muscle groups, *e.g.* shoulder adductors, elbow and wrist flexors.

The clinical picture was summarized by Walshe (1923) and attributed to unsuppressed input from the otoliths of the inner ear and neck proprioceptors.

The importance of inputs from the labyrinths must not be overlooked since they determine much of the inappropriate posturing in so-called 'spastic hemiplegia' and 'spastic diplegia': such excessive tonic labyrinthine input interferes enormously with voluntary movement while varying exquisitely with the position of the head in space and nonspecific afferent inputs (emotions, hunger, pain, intellectual activity), all of which alter the level of arousal.

iv. Tonic labyrinthine input and dorsal rhizotomy

An important physiological observation was made by Denny-Brown who noted that in earlier work with primates, dorsal rhizotomy failed to abolish the tonic labyrinthine response (Denny-Brown and Bottrell 1947; Denny-Brown 1966, 1980).

v. Sleep and postures sustained by tonic labyrinthine inputs

Sleep abolishes these labyrinthine-dependent postures. Dystonic postures along with all parkinsonian rigidity, tics, chorea and athetosis, are always abolished by sleep irrespective of cause (Fish *et al.* 1991). The effect of deep sleep on the child (or adult) should always be recorded; indeed, achieving a good night's sleep should be a focus of the management plan. Good sleep may significantly relieve night cramps and spasms and may reduce the rate of progression of contractures through limb relaxation (Lin 1998). However, if the underlying muscle stiffness is intrinsic to the muscles and not supported by supraspinal mechanisms, children may in fact wake up more stiffly in the morning because of reduced movements at night.

vi. Posture and deformity

Abnormally sustained and stereotyped postures eventually result in permanent deformity through contracture of muscles unless the body is able to move through a wide range of postures or to relax for considerable periods each day: *postures, not spasticity, produce deformity*.

SPASTICITY AND REFLEX EXCITABILITY

Spasticity: what is it, what is it not?

One of the major obstacles to management has been in the definition and interpretation of the term 'spasticity', inherent in the classification of the dominant form of the cerebral palsies (Surveillance of Cerebral Palsy in Europe 2002). The 'treatment of spasticity' may occupy a disproportionately large part of the overall management programme. Because of this, the

TABLE 7.1
Syndromic spasticity*

1. Muscular hypertonus of the clasp-knife type
2. Hyperreflexia, which is further usually of constant duplicable degree on repeated elicitation
3. Positive Babinski and Hoffman reflexes, although the latter is probably an exaggeration and overflow of the finger jerk rather than a 'pyramidal-tract sign'
4. Diminished superficial reflexes (abdominal and cremasteric)
5. Release of postural and labyrinthine reflexes
6. Spread and overflow of associated movements
7. Loss of voluntary control of fine movements
8. Frequently clonus of the ankle or other joints, although this is not at all universal or essential
9. A tendency to muscular contracture in characteristic postures

*Adapted from Crothers and Paine (1959).

TABLE 7.2
Possible interpretations of the term 'spasticity'*

Definition	Possible interpretation
Proprioceptive reflex release	Unstimulated muscle is quiescent, with increased phasic and tonic stretch reflexes and a clasp-knife response
Generalised reflex release chronic paraplegia	Including polysynaptic flexion reflexes, *e.g.* chronic flexor spasms of
Upper motor neuron syndrome	Poor motor performance and reflex release
Dystonic-rigid state	Ill-defined with many causes and pathological features, characterized by continuous muscle contraction: so-called 'busy line'
Mixed	Combinations of 1–4
Undefined	

*Adapted by permission from Landau (1974).

bulk of this chapter must necessarily be devoted to the pathophysiology of disordered muscle tone, during the course of which it will be seen that 'spasticity' in fact represents a minor part of the totality of the motor disorder. Accordingly, it will be argued that there is no such thing as a 'spastic posture' or a 'spastic muscle'.

Definitions of spasticity and the spastic syndrome
There have been varying interpretations of the meaning of spasticity over the past century. Crothers and Paine (1959) defined spasticity as a clinical spectrum of motor manifestations (*i.e.* a syndromic definition, Table 7.1). Landau (1974) looked critically at a number of prevailing 'definitions' of spasticity (Table 7.2) with a view to highlighting the lack of clinical and scientific rigour in the existing definitions. Looking at these two tables one might wonder how one could measure spasticity according to these definitions, since the definitions include so many different aspects of motor dysfunction?

Measurement of spasticity
The currently accepted physiological definition was enunciated by Lance (1980): "In both cerebral and spinal spasticity, the stretch reflex responses obtainable from extensor and flexor

93

muscle groups of the upper and lower limbs increases approximately linearly with the increase in the velocity of stretch. The reflex component of the increased tone may therefore be measured in terms of the threshold velocity required to evoke reflex activity and the slope of the EMG–velocity relationship."

Such velocity-dependent increases in reflex excitability are secondary to damaged or lost supraspinal inputs (due to reduced presynaptic inhibition) and may be observed, measured and reduced through medical intervention *if clinically significant* (Crenna *et al.* 1992, Lin *et al.* 1994a). Establishing the clinical significance of spasticity, though desirable, is only rarely practised. It is seldom useful to reduce reflex excitability at the expense of reduced truncal control, increased sedation or excessive drooling. It is also seldom helpful to administer oral muscle relaxants in children and adults with hemisyndromes because of unwanted systemic effects. On the other hand, genuine bilateral spasticity may produce very disabling symptoms such as velocity-dependent increases in quadriceps and plantarflexor muscle activity that interfere with flexion of the knee and clearance of the foot in the swing phase of gait or in climbing stairs, or may infrequently be associated with severe, disabling clonus that interferes with standing. The interference with lower and upper limb function by spasticity has been questioned. McLellan (1977) was unable to suppress co-contraction in quadriceps and hamstring muscles with oral baclofen, despite the fact that the velocity-dependent stretch reflexes were reduced by the treatment. During isometric force tracking tasks, abnormal elbow flexor muscle peak EMG discharges occurred in the absence of an extensor movement capable of provoking a reflex discharge (McClellan *et al.* 1985), resulting in the conclusion that these discharges were attributable to abnormal motor planning, not to spasticity (however, see section on intrathecal baclofen, pp. 98–99).

By definition, there can be no such thing as a 'spastic posture' (Burke 1988), since the posture, being sustained, is not supported by a velocity stimulus. Likewise, there is no such thing as 'spastic muscle'.

The natural history of spasticity
In any individual, spasticity will vary according to the state of arousal as well as according to the time that has elapsed since the cerebral injury. Herman (1970) documented the natural history of reflex excitability in the aftermath of acute stroke, identifying four phases:
Phase I: Flaccid and inexcitable
Phase II: Hyperreflexia and clonus in the first few months, lasting a few years
Phase III: Reduction in reflex excitability
Phase IV: Stiff, inexcitable and shortened muscles: fixed contracture.

This scheme suggested that the properties of muscles determined in part the excitability of the system. In phase I, although the system is greatly under-damped (flaccid) the velocity-dependent stretch reflexes may not be markedly brisk. During stage II, the muscles are not intrinsically stiff, but the reflex velocity threshold is lower than normal due to loss of presynaptic inhibition: spasticity may be unbridled. By the time phases III and IV are reached, the muscles are getting stiffer and it becomes physically difficult to stretch them rapidly. Accordingly, the reflex velocity threshold cannot be reached. By the same token, as muscle properties alter towards contracture, so the angle at which maximum reflex excitability is elicited changes, thus altering the joint-angle–reflex-excitability curve (Lin *et al*. 1999).

MUSCULAR TRANSFORMATION AND CONTRACTURE: SERIAL CASTING AND SOFT-TISSUE SURGERY

This section deals with aspects of muscle tone that are independent of the electrical excitation of muscle.

Visco-elastic properties of muscle

Muscles resist stretching in several ways. There is length-dependent resistance, called elasticity. Muscles also exhibit viscous properties, viscous resistance increasing in proportion to the speed of stretch (imagine dragging a spoon through honey or attempting to walk rapidly in a swimming pool: the resistance encountered rises as the speed of motion increases, representing viscous drag). Changes in these visco-elastic properties have been documented following stroke in adults (Hufschmidt and Mauritz 1985) and in children (Dietz *et al*. 1981, Dietz and Berger 1995). Accordingly, the work required to stretch such transformed muscles increases (this is seen as an absorption power graph in gait laboratory reports). Progressive collagen accumulation has been found in muscles of children with CP (Booth *et al*. 2001), supporting the view of muscles tending to a fibro-fatty, ligneous (woody) inexcitable state over time.

Muscles thus may become stiffer (less compliant) owing to rheological changes in the muscle tissue itself. This stiffness is not dependent on muscle depolarization and cannot be reversed with muscle relaxants. Contractures are posture-dependent and arise through disuse and weakness. The risk of multilevel contractures increases with age as bone growth outstrips muscle growth.

The relationship between muscle length and muscle tension

There is no muscle length without tension. Examination of a piece of muscle (*e.g.* fresh meat) reveals a soft, sticky material that is devoid of tension when probed. Muscle *in situ* behaves differently. In fact, the tension and length vary with the joint angle and vice versa. Most of us are familiar with the principle of the stringed instrument, which is tuned by varying the tension and the length of the string to be plucked or hit. The longer the string and the lower the tension, the lower the note and the lower the resonant frequency. The shorter the string and the higher the tension, the higher the note and the higher the resonant frequency. The 'resonant frequency' is defined as the frequency at which the amplitude of motion of the string (or object) is maximal: such frequencies can be obtained in children at any joint. The resonant frequency is also inversely proportional to the inertia of the limb. Resonant frequency (RF) is thus a measure of muscle stiffness and limb inertia. Different limbs and muscles resonate at different frequencies, reflecting differences in length and tension in the muscles and varying according to the joint angle of any specified limb (flexion–extension; abduction–adduction). In addition to variations in passive muscle stiffness with joint angle, long limbs have high inertia, which will reduce the resonant frequency obtained (Table 7.3). Short limbs such as digits have little inertia and as such might be expected to vibrate or

TABLE 7.3
Resonant frequencies at different joints in healthy adult subjects: relationship between stiffness and inertia of limb

Joint	Plane of motion	Resonant frequency	Stiffness relative to elbow joint
Hip	Abduction–adduction	0.5	1
Hip	Axial rotation	4.0	8
Knee	Flexion–extension	0.5	1
Ankle	Dorsiflexion–plantraflexion	5.0	10
Elbow	Flexion–extension	0.5	1
Wrist	Flexion–extension	2.5	5
MCPJ	Flexion–extension	20.0	40

Note the extreme stiffness of the metacarpophalangeal joints (MCPJ).

There is an inverse relationship between limb inertia and muscle stiffness. Since inertia resists motion, large limbs require little by way of muscle stiffness to dampen movements. Small limbs, particularly digits, have little inertia but their muscles compensate with increased stiffness.

$$RF = \frac{1\sqrt{K/J}}{2\pi} \quad \text{and} \quad K = \frac{(2\pi RF)^2}{J}$$

According to this relationship, the stiffness (K) will vary according the square of the resonant frequency (RF) multiplied by 2π and divided by the inertia (J). Assuming the inertia to be constant for any given limb, a doubling in RF implies a 24-fold increase in muscle stiffness. Small changes in RF are caused by large changes in stiffness. With growth of the limb, inertia and stiffness contribute to the resistance to motion.

shake when the subject is walking, running, jumping or throwing. However, the muscles acting across the joints of small digits are exceptionally stiff so that the RF at the metacarpophalangeal joint (MCPJ) is 40 times greater than the RF of muscles acting at the hip or knee (Table 7.3).

Range of stiffness with passive stretching
When muscles are passively stretched, the tension rises and the RF rises. Passively stretching muscles requires an external force (moment). A massive (60–250%) increase in muscle stiffness occurs as the calf muscles of children with diplegia are stretched using a 'standing torque' for any given sinusoidal 'driving (applied) torque' (personal data, unpublished). There is also a corresponding dramatic reduction in the maximum amplitude of motion at resonance for any given driving torque with increasing standing torque.

Active (dynamic) and passive muscle stiffness
Changes in RF are a sensitive marker of changes in muscle stiffness, since the inertial properties of the limbs are constant in the short term. If a frequency–amplitude graph is plotted for the ankle, multiple resonant frequency peaks at different frequencies can be demonstrated. These are abolished by diazepam. Diazepam abolishes the reflex perturbations, which are now replaced by a smooth chirp outline. However, the post-diazepam resonant frequency may be higher by almost 2 Hz than the peak resonance associated with peak displacement pre-diazepam (personal data, unpublished). This apparent paradox may be

explained by the fact that muscles that twitch may be intrinsically looser than muscles that do not, because twitches maintain muscles in a semi-fluid state, *i.e.* they alter the thixotropic properties of the underlying muscles (Lakie *et al.* 1984, Walsh 1992). Muscles which have recently moved are intrinsically less stiff than muscles which have been immobile. Diazepam can thus be said to unmask the underlying increased stiffness of the calf in diplegia.

Peripheral alterations in muscle properties and reflex excitability with surgery or casting

Herman's studies in the 1970s indicated that muscle properties and the degree of reflex excitability were interconnected. Moreover, the resistance to passive stretching changed as the time from the cerebral injury elapsed (see above). Lin and coworkers (Lin and Brown 1992; Lin *et al.* 1996b, 1997, 1999; Lin 1998) obtained direct confirmation of these central and peripheral interactions. An exploration of the reflex excitability of the soleus stretch reflex in children with hemiplegic CP revealed that the reflex was greatest in amplitude in relatively under-damped muscles (Lin 1998, Lin *et al.* 1999). There was a close link between the contractile properties of the muscles and reflex excitability, once again yoking the neurophysiology to intramuscular changes. Accordingly, the reflex EMG amplitude was greatest in hemiparetic limbs that exhibited clonus to rapid muscular stretching. However, for hemiparetic limbs that did not exhibit clonus (*i.e.* the majority of limbs) the duration of the reflex muscle twitch, and the half contraction and half relaxation times, were significantly longer than in limbs exhibiting clonus and in healthy control muscles (Lin *et al.* 1999). The authors hypothesized that the history of muscle activity for any given limb alters the mechanical properties of the muscle and thus influences the reflex excitability of the system. Relief from contracture may be achieved with plaster immobilization under moderate tension such as 'serial casting' at progressively increased joint angles, with an inevitable change in the mechanical properties of the muscles and reflex excitability (muscle loading, Lin *et al.* 1999).

Soft-tissue releases (muscle unloading) may also result in increased reflex excitability (clonus) that decreases with time (Lin *et al.* 1999). Alterations in the muscle properties following casting or surgery may thus alter the expression of spinal reflex excitability and the physiology of clonus (Lin *et al.* 1999). These procedures have the effect of under-damping muscles. There is no evidence to suggest that casting for a period 'inhibits' muscle tone, though plenty of data to confirm the advent of muscle wasting. At the other end of the spectrum, complete unloading of a muscle results in an almost areflexic, flaccid state (Vrbová 1963).

Management of specific aspects of 'muscle hypertonus'

The first aim is to manage the expectations and specific goals of the child, family and re-ferring team, by working towards commonly agreed goals. We have already seen strategies for monitoring and potentially altering a wide range of motor phenomena: some of these phenomena are due to the passive (EMG-negative) intrinsic properties of limbs, while others are secondary to muscle activation (EMG-positive).

Strategies may be directed to the 'whole body' at one end of the spectrum, to the disordered limb or muscle function at the other, or both. Total body approaches tend to be aimed at nonspecific improvements in well-being of the child, whereas focal strategies usually have specific goals, for instance the management of equinus, fisting or spasms.

WHOLE BODY APPROACHES
General care
The most widely used management should be attention to feeding and nutrition, posture and seating, sleep pattern and psychological contentment (*i.e.* the reduction of frustration in all its various manifestations). As the discussion on the mechanisms of disordered muscle tone have demonstrated, nonspecific entities affecting the state of arousal such as pain, irritability, fatigue and frustration play an enormous role in exacerbating disordered motor function. Relief from the pain of gastro-oesaphageal reflux, hip dysplasia/dislocation, dental caries, pressure sores and nocturnal spasms should be actively explored. Where sleep is significantly disordered, restoration of adequately deep sleep should be actively explored, since sleep has such a profound effect on reducing abnormal muscle tone. Although there are many sedative preparations with varying muscle-relaxing properties, melatonin, a naturally occurring 'sleep hormone', has proven to be an excellent means of promoting the initiation of sleep in children with CP and other disabilities (Ross *et al.* 2002).

Oral medication
A mainstay of all programmes of care has been the judicial use of oral medication such as baclofen, benzodiazepines (diazepam, nitrazepam), dantrolene (an intramuscular calcium re-uptake inhibitor) and tizanidine (alpha-adrenergic blockers). In the majority of cases, these oral medications have been aimed at relieving varying forms of sustained muscle over-activity (*i.e.* rigidity) or troublesome (painful) spasms. Treatment has to be titrated against troublesome systemic effects such as truncal floppiness, somnolence, poor concentration and drooling. These unwanted effects often limit the usefulness of systemic medication, particularly as limb stiffness and rigidity often persist despite truncal floppiness. This is in part because not all limb-joint stiffness is attributable to active muscular contraction (see above), and the Ashworth Scale cannot differentiate between active and passive resistance to stretch (Damiano *et al.* 2002). Recently, further studies comparing H-reflex to M-response ratios to the Modified Ashworth Scale (MAS) elicited at the ankle in post-stroke adults suggests that the MAS is more a measure of hypertonia rather than spasticity (Bakheit *et al.* 2003).

Intrathecal baclofen
This can be considered as a whole-body management strategy with a gradient for the lower trunk and legs, owing to the physical settling of the instilled baclofen in the lower cerebrospinal fluid.

There are some striking examples of physiological improvement in function following the use of intrathecal baclofen (ITB) infusions (Penn 1988). These include relief of co-contraction; abolition of unwanted muscle coactivation during voluntary tasks without reduction of the desired voluntary muscle EMG output; and relief from excessive reflex excitability such as clonus of the antagonist muscle (Latash *et al.* 1990).

The literature on the evidence for the efficacy of ITB in CP has been exhaustively reviewed by a committee of the American Academy of Cerebral Palsy and Developmental Medicine (Butler and Campbell 2000). Case series have suggested symptomatic relief of distressing spasms based on assessments of reductions on the Ashworth Scale for spasticity (Albright *et al.* 1991) and the possibility of prevention of intramuscular contractures or the need for orthopaedic procedures (Gerzetsen *et al.* 1998). Despite early reports that ITB was unsuitable in children with dystonia (Albright *et al.* 1991), subsequent studies have indicated its effectiveness (Albright *et al.* 2001). This modality has traditionally been reserved for children with total body involvement and has been shown to be safe and well tolerated over time (Campbell *et al.* 2002). However, despite improvements in ease of comfort and high parent/carer satisfaction, the same study failed to demonstrate improvements in the Gross Motor Function Measure (GMFM: Russell *et al.* 1989, 2002) over the same period for these severely motor-impaired children. Because ITB reduces both spasticity and dystonia, it is inappropriate to use the efficacy of reduced tone with ITB as a means of selecting children for dorsal rhizotomy (see below). Sound neuroanatomical reasons for the mode of action of continuous ITB in dystonia have been advanced (Lin 2000) based on the distribution of GABA-B receptors deep in the spinal cord. Time to penetrate to deeper layers to reach GABA-B receptors on the presynaptic terminals of supraspinal fibres is one mechanism by which ITB exerts an antidystonic effect.

Dorsal rhizotomy
Strictly speaking, rhizotomy is a regional therapeutic modality, usually directed to relieving leg spasticity and improving leg function. Much has been written about this procedure, which has had wide exposure in children with CP, particularly in North America. Two randomized studies of ITB plus intensive physiotherapy in Canada (Steinbok *et al.* 1997, Wright *et al.* 1998) indicated improvements in GMFM scores and reductions in the Ashworth score when compared with intensive physiotherapy alone. A third study from the USA, although clearly demonstrating reduced spasticity (by instrumented measures of assessment) could not clearly show a superiority of dorsal rhizotomy over intensive strengthening exercises, although older case selection, division of fewer dorsal rootlets and a more aggressive physiotherapy programme in the 'non-intervention group' were features of this study (McLaughlin *et al.* 1998). A meta-analysis of these three studies did fall narrowly in favour of a 4% increase in GMFM in children receiving dorsal rhizotomy (McLaughlin *et al.* 2002). It is important to state at this juncture that the intra-operative nerve root selection procedure has been seriously called into question (Hays *et al.* 1998), suggesting that the procedure might more aptly be termed 'partial dorsal rhizotomy'.

FOCAL MANAGEMENT STRATEGIES: BOTULINUM TOXIN A
There has been an explosion of interest in the use of botulinum toxin A (BTX-A) in children with CP since it was first used to manage squints in 1981. Several books have now covered the topic extensively and provide detailed information about indications for use, dosage and site of injection (Neville and Albright 2000, Barnes and Johnson 2002, Moore and Naumann 2003). In most countries, the only licensed indication for BTX-A use in

children is for the relief of dynamic equinus, other indications being the responsibility of the clinician.

An important caveat accompanies all publications in this field, namely the difference in potency between Botox (Allergan) and Dysport (Ipsen), as, unit for unit, Botox is approximately three times as potent as Dysport. Most studies have focussed on the effects of BTX-A on the legs, and the majority of these have been open-labelled studies. However, larger randomized, double-blind, placebo-controlled dose-ranging studies of safety and efficacy of BTX-A are now available for scrutiny. The effects of varying doses of Dysport compared with placebo were studied in 120 diplegic children (Baker *et al*. 2002). This study demonstrated an optimal response in reducing dynamic equinus when calf muscles received 20 units/kg body weight as opposed to placebo, 10 units/kg or 30 units/kg. However, the GMFM was not significantly improved by any dose. A study of 48 children aged 3–15 years (mean 7 years 6 months) with hemiplegic CP involved a double-blind, randomized comparison of two doses of BTX-A (Dysport); 24 units/kg and 8 units/kg body weight (Polak *et al*. 2002), maximum improvement occurring in children receiving the higher dose when judged according to sagittal plane joint kinematics using gait analysis. The superiority of the higher dose resulted in the absolute dose falling to between 200 and 500 units of Dysport per calf muscle.

The relationship between the dosage per kilogram and dose per muscle remains largely unresolved. A maximum dose of Dysport of 1000 units per injection course has been recommended (Bakheit *et al*. 2001) to reduce the risk of side-effects (11% of cases) with higher doses (22% of cases). Most of the reported side-effects were minor. Further advice on dosage for either Botox or Dysport for specific muscles in children is given by Berwick *et al*. (2003). *The Management of Adults with Spasticity Using Botulinum Toxin: a Guide to Clinical Practice* (2001) (available from Radius Healthcare, Suite 2, Cobb House, Oyster Lane, Byfleet, Surrey KT14 7DU, England) is a well-referenced consensus document containing useful discussion of specific indications, dosage charts and assessment forms for use in adults, but nevertheless generalizable to adolescents.

The histological effects on the muscles of rabbits of BTX-A toxin dose, toxin dilution and muscle stretching exercises have recently been reported (Kim *et al*. 2003). Higher doses and higher dilutions along with a stretching programme produce the greatest histological changes of atrophy. These effects are not unlike the effects of soft-tissue surgical releases demonstrated in healthy rabbits (Cotter and Phillips 1986, Cotter *et al*. 1988), except that mechanical stimulation of toxin-injected muscles accentuates the atrophy, whereas electrical stimulation of tenotomized muscles results in restoration of normal muscle histology.

COMBINED MANAGEMENT STRATEGIES
There is still a great deal of division within the field between proponents of neurodevelopmental 'treatments' and those who favour specific physical intervention techniques. A general benefit to the field of CP management has been the increased level of rigour and scientific scrutiny of levels of evidence for efficacy of treatments. An outstanding review of neurodevelopmental intervention programmes spanning the years 1990–2001 (Siebes *et*

al. 2002) indicates that fundamental research with adequate methodology was applied more frequently than in the period 1980–1989, but that these developments had not led to a substantial improvement in the scientific foundation of the interventions under study. The authors conclude: "single case studies, combined with efforts to develop measures specifically for children with CP and with high sensitivity, might make more valuable contributions to the scientific justification for therapeutic intervention."

In practice, as is amply evident from the titles in this book, and the contents of this chapter, no specific therapeutic instrument is used in isolation. Rather, combinations are harnessed to produce maximum benefit to posture and mobility, including strength training, orthotics, and single and multilevel surgery. The aims, as always, are to address primary dysfunction, not the compensatory mechanisms, though many parents will interpret removing the latter among their goals.

Muscle tone is a complex physiological amalgam of different physiological processes. Different aspects may be selected for intervention provided clear goals and objectives are established at the outset. Successful attainment of the goals thus validates the intervention.

REFERENCES

Albright, A.L., Cervi, A., Singletary, J. (1991) 'Intrathecal baclofen for spasticity in cerebral palsy.' *Journal of the American Medical Association*, **265**, 1418–1422.

Albright, A.L., Barry, M.J., Shafron, D.H., Ferson, S.S. (2001) 'Intrathecal baclofen for generalized dystonia.' *Developmental Medicine and Child Neurology*, **43**, 652–657.

Anslow, P. (2002) 'Radiological assessment of the child with cerebral palsy and its medicolegal implications.' *In:* Squier, W. (Ed.) *Acquired Damage to the Developing Brain.* London: Arnold, pp. 166–192.

Baker, R., Jasinski, M., Maciag-Tymecka, I., Michalowska-Mrozek, J., Bonikowski, M., Carr, L., Maclean, J., Lin, J-P., Lynch, B., Theologis, T., Wendorff, J., Eunson, P., Cosgrove, A. (2002) 'Botulinum toxin treatment of spasticity in diplegic cerebral palsy: a randomized, double-blind, placebo-controlled, dose-ranging study.' *Developmental Medicine and Child Neurology*, **44**, 666–675.

Bakheit, A.M.O., Severa, S., Cosgrove, A., Morton, R., Roussounis, S.H., Doderlein, L., Lin, J-P. (2001) 'Safety profile and efficacy of botulinum toxin A (Dysport) in children with muscle spasticity.' *Developmental Medicine and Child Neurology*, **43**, 234–238.

Bakheit, A.M.O., Maynard, V.A., Curnow, J., Hudson, N., Kodapala, S. (2003) 'The relation between Ashworth scale scores and the excitability of the alpha-motor neurones in patients with post-stroke muscle spasticity.' *Journal of Neurology, Neurosurgery and Psychiatry*, **74**, 646–648.

Barnes, M.P., Johnson, G.R. (Eds.) (2001) *Upper Motor Syndrome and Spasticity: Clinical Management and Neurophysiology.* Cambridge: Cambridge University Press.

Berwick, S., Graham, H.K., Heinen, F. (2003) 'Spasticity in children.' *In:* Moore, P., Nauman, M. (Eds.) *Handbook of Botulinum Toxin Treatment, 2nd Edn.* Oxford: Blackwell Science, pp. 272–303.

Booth, C.M., Cortina-Borja, M.J., Theologis, T.N. (2001) 'Collagen accumulation in muscles of children with cerebral palsy and correlation with severity of spasticity.' *Developmental Medicine and Child Neurology*, **43**, 314–320.

Brown, J.K., Omar, T., O'Regan, M. (1997) 'Brain development and the development of tone and movement.' *In:* Connolly, K., Forssberg, H. (Eds.) *Neurophysiology and Neuropsychology of Motor Development. Clinics in Developmental Medicine No. 143–144.* London: Mac Keith Press, pp. 1–41.

Burke, D. (1988) 'Spasticity as an adaptation to pyramidal tract injury.' *Advances in Neurology*, **47**, 401–423.

Butler, C., Campbell, S. (2000) 'Evidence of the effects of intrathecal baclofen for spastic and dystonic cerebral palsy.' *Developmental Medicine and Child Neurology*, **42**, 634–645.

Campbell, W.M., Ferrell, A., McLaughlin, J.F., Grant, G.A., Loeser, J.D., Graubert, C., Bjornson, K. (2002) 'Long-term safety and efficacy of continuous intrathecal baclofen.' *Developmental Medicine and Child Neurology*, **44**, 660–665.

Christensen, E., Melchior, J. (1967) *Cerebral Palsy. A Clinical and Neuropathological Study. Clinics in*

Developmental Medicine No. 25. London: Spastics Society Medical Education and Information Unit.

Cotter, M., Phillips, P. (1986) 'Rapid fast to slow fiber transformation in response to chronic stimulation of immobilized muscle of the rabbit.' *Experimental Neurology*, **93**, 531–545.

Cotter, M.A., Barry, J.A., Cameron, N.E. (1988) 'Recovery from immobilization-induced atrophy of rabbit soleus muscles can be accelerated by chronic low-frequency stimulation.' *Quarterly Journal of Experimental Physiology*, **73**, 797–800.

Crenna, P., Inverno, M., Frigo, C., Palmieri, R., Fedrizzi, E. (1992) 'Pathophysiological profile of gait in children with cerebral palsy.' *In:* Forssberg, H., Hirschfeld, H. (Eds.) *Movement Disorders in Children. Medicine and Sport Science, Vol. 36.* Basel: Karger, pp. 186–198.

Crothers, B., Paine, R.S. (1959) *The Natural History of Cerebral Palsy.* (Reprinted as *Classics in Developmental Medicine No. 2.* Mac Keith Press, London, 1988.)

Damiano, D.L., Quinlivan, J.M., Owen, B.F., Payne, P., Nelson, K.C., Abel, M.F. (2002) 'What does the Ashworth Scale really measure and are instrumented measures more valid and precise?' *Developmental Medicine and Child Neurology*, **44**, 112–118.

Denny-Brown, D. (1966) *The Cerebral Control of Movement.* Liverpool: Liverpool University Press.

Denny-Brown, D. (1980) 'Historical aspects of the relation of spasticity to movement.' *In:* Feldman, R.G., Young, R.R., Koella, W.P. (Eds.) *Spasticity: Disordered Motor Control.* Chicago: Year Book Publishers, pp. 1–15.

Denny-Brown, D., Bottrell, E.H. (1947) 'The motor functions of the agranular frontal cortex.' *Research Publications of the Association for Nervous and Medical Disorders*, **27**, 2235–2345.

Detrembleur, C., Willems, P., Plaghki, L. (1997) 'Does walking speed influence the time pattern of muscle activation in normal children?' *Developmental Medicine and Child Neurology*, **39**, 803–807.

Dietz, V., Berger, W. (1995) 'Cerebral palsy and muscle transformation.' *Developmental Medicine and Child Neurology*, **37**, 180–184.

Dietz, V., Quintern, J., Berger, W. (1981) 'Electrophysiological studies of gait in spasticity and rigidity: evidence that altered mechanical properties of muscle contribute to hypertonia.' *Brain*, **104**, 431–449.

Evarts, E.V. (1968) 'Relation of pyramidal tract activity to force exerted during voluntary movement.' *Journal of Neurophysiology*, **31**, 14–27.

Fish, D.R., Sawyers, D., Allen, P.J., Blackie, J.D., Lees, A.J., Marsden, C.D. (1991) 'The effect of sleep on the dyskinetic movements of Parkinson's disease, Gilles de la Tourette syndrome, Huntington's disease and torsion dystonia.' *Archives of Neurology*, **48**, 210–214.

Føg, E., Føg, M. (1963) 'Cerebral inhibition examined by associated movements.' *In:* Bax, M., Mac Keith, R. (Eds.) *Minimal Cerebral Dysfunction. Clinics in Developmental Medicine No. 10.* London: Spastics International Medical Publications, pp. 52–57.

Freud, S. (1897) 'Die infantile Cerebrallahmung.' *In:* Nothnagel. H. (Ed.) *Specielle Pathologie und Therapie. Vol. 9, No. 3.* Vienna: Alfred Holder.

Gerzertsen, P.C., Albright, A.L., Johnstone, G.E. (1998) 'Intrathecal baclofen infusion and subsequent orthopaedic surgery in patients with spastic cerebral palsy.' *Journal of Neurosurgery*, **88**, 1009–1013.

Hays, R.M., McLaughlin, J.F., Bjornson, K.F., Stephens, K., Roberts, T.S., Price, R. (1998) 'Electrophysiological monitoring during selective dorsal rhizotomy, and spasticity and GMFM performance.' *Developmental Medicine and Child Neurology*, **40**, 233–238.

Herman, R. (1970) 'The myotatic reflex: clinico-physiological aspects of spasticity and contracture.' *Brain*, **93**, 273–312.

Hufschmidt, A., Mauritz, K-H. (1985) 'Chronic transformation of muscle in spasticity: a peripheral contribution to increased tone.' *Journal of Neurology, Neurosurgery, and Psychiatry*, **48**, 676–685.

Kim, H.S., Hwang, J.H., Jeong, S.T., Lee, Y.T., Suh, Y-L., Shim, J.S. (2003) 'Effect of muscle activity and botulinum toxin dilution volume on muscle paralysis.' *Developmental Medicine and Child Neurology*, **45**, 200–205.

Krageloh-Mann, I. (2000) 'Magnetic resonance imaging in cerebral palsy.' *In:* Neville, B., Albright, A.L. (Eds.) *The Management of Spasticity Associated with the Cerebral Palsies in Children and Adolescents.* Secaucus, NJ: Churchill Communications, pp. 52–61.

Lakie, M., Walsh, E.G., Wright, G.W. (1984) 'Resonance at the wrist demonstrated by the use of a torque motor, an instrumental analysis of muscle tone in man.' *Journal of Physiology*, **353**, 265–285.

Lance, J.W. (1980) 'Pathophysiology of spasticity and clinical experience with baclofen.' *In:* Feldman, R.G., Young, R.R., Koella, W.P. (Eds.) *Spasticity: Disordered Motor Control.* Chicago: Year Book Medical Publishers, pp. 185–203.

Landau, W. (1974) 'Spasticity: the fable of the neurological demon and the Emperor's new therapy.' *Archives of Neurology*, **31**, 217–219.

Latash, M.L., Penn, R.D., Corcos, D.M., Gottlieb, G.L. (1990) 'Effects of intrathecal baclofen on voluntary motor control in spastic paresis.' *Journal of Neurosurgery*, **72**, 388–392.

Leonard, C.T., Hirschfeld, H., Forssberg, H. (1991) 'The development of independent walking in children with cerebral palsy.' *Developmental Medicine and Child Neurology*, **33**, 567–577.

Lin, J-P. (1998) 'Motor assessments in cerebral palsy: a study of the mechanisms of equinus, the functional neuromuscular angle, clonus, alternating movements and posture.' Ph.D. thesis, University of Edinburgh, Faculty of Medicine.

Lin, J-P. (2000) 'The pathophysiology of spasticity and dystonia.' *In:* Neville, B., Albright, A.L. (Eds.) *The Management of Spasticity Associated with the Cerebral Palsies in Children and Adolescents*. Secaucus, NJ: Churchill Communications, pp. 11–38.

Lin, J-P. (2003) 'The cerebral palsies: a physiological approach.' *Journal of Neurology, Neurosurgery, and Psychiatry*, Suppl. 1, i23–i29.

Lin, J-P., Brown, J.K. (1992) 'Peripheral and central mechanisms of hindfoot equinus in childhood hemiplegia.' *Developmental Medicine and Child Neurology*, **34**, 662–670.

Lin, J-P., Brown, J.K., Brotherstone, R. (1994a) 'Assessment of spasticity in hemiplegic cerebral palsy. II. Distal lower-limb reflex excitability.' *Developmental Medicine and Child Neurology*, **36**, 290–303.

Lin, J-P., Brown, J.K., Walsh, E.G. (1994b) 'Physiological maturation of muscles in childhood.' *Lancet*, **343**, 1386–1389.

Lin, J-P., Brown, J.K., Walsh, E.G. (1996a) 'The maturation of motor dexterity: or why Johnny can't go any faster.' *Developmental Medicine and Child Neurology*, **38**, 244–254.

Lin, J-P., Brown, J.K., Walsh, E.G. (1996b) 'Joint angle modulation of reflex neuromuscular output at the ankle in man.' *Journal of Physiology*, **495**, 148P.

Lin, J-P., Brown, J.K., Walsh, E.G. (1997) 'Soleus muscle length, stretch reflex excitability and the contractile properties of muscle in children and adults: a study of the functional joint angle.' *Developmental Medicine and Child Neurology*, **39**, 469–480.

Lin, J-P., Brown, J.K., Walsh, E.G. (1999) 'The continuum of reflex excitability in hemiplegia: influence of muscle length and muscular transformation after heel-cord lengthening and immobilization on the pathophysiology of spasticity and clonus.' *Developmental Medicine and Child Neurology*, **41**, 534–548.

McLaughlin, J.F., Bjornson, K.F., Astley, S.J., Graubert, C., Hays, R.M., Roberts, T.S., Price, R., Temkin, N. (1998) 'Selective dorsal rhizotomy: efficacy and safety in an investigator-masked randomized clinical trial.' *Developmental Medicine and Child Neurology*, **40**, 220–232.

McLaughlin, J., Bjornson, K., Temkin, N., Steinbok, P., Wright, V., Reiner, A., Roberts, T.S., Drake, J., O'Donnell, M., Rosenbaum, P., Barber, J., Ferrel, A. (2002) 'Selective dorsal rhizotomy: meta-analysis of three randomized controlled trials.' *Developmental Medicine and Child Neurology*, **44**, 17–25.

McLellan, D.L. (1977) 'Co-contraction and stretch reflexes in spasticity during treatment with baclofen.' *Journal of Neurology, Neurosurgery, and Psychiatry*, **40**, 30–38.

McLellan, D.L., Hassan, N., Hodgson, J.A. (1985) 'Tracking tasks in the assessment of spasticity.' *In:* Delwaide, P., Young, R.R. (Eds.) *Clinical Neurophysiology in Spasticity*. Amsterdam: Elsevier Science, pp. 131–139.

Moore, P., Naumann, M. (Eds.) (2003) *Handbook of Botulinum Toxin Treatment, 2nd Edn*. Oxford: Blackwell Science.

Mutch, L., Alberman, E., Hagberg, B., Kodama, K., Perat, M.V. (1992) 'Cerebral palsy epidemiology: where are we now and where are we going?' *Developmental Medicine and Child Neurology*, **34**, 547–555.

Nashner, L.M. (1985) 'A functional approach to understanding spasticity.' *In:* Struppler, A., Weindl, A. (Eds.) *Electromyography and Evoked Potentials*. Berlin: Springer-Verlag, pp. 22–29.

Nashner, L.M., Shumway, A., Marin, O. (1983) 'Stance posture and control in selected groups of children with cerebral palsy: deficits in sensory integration and muscular coordination.' *Experimental Brain Research*, **49**, 393–409.

Nelson, K.B., Ellenberg, J.H. (1982) 'Children who 'outgrew' cerebral palsy.' *Pediatrics*, **69**, 529–536.

Neville, B., Albright, A.L. (Eds.) (2000) *The Management of Spasticity Associated with the Cerebral Palsies in Children and Adolescents*. Secaucus, NJ: Churchill Communications.

Osler, W. (1889) *The Cerebral Palsies of Children*. (Reprinted as *Classics in Developmental Medicine No. 1*. Mac Keith Press, London, 1987.)

Penn, R.D. (1988) 'Intrathecal baclofen for severe spasticity.' *Annals of the New York Academy of Sciences*, **531**, 157–166.

Polak, F., Morton, R., Ward, C., Wallace, A., Doderlein, L., Siebel, A. (2002) 'Double-blind comparison study of two doses of botulinum toxin A injected into calf muscles in children with hemiplegic cerebral palsy.' *Developmental Medicine and Child Neurology*, **44**, 551–555.

Ross, C., Davies, P., Whitehouse, W. (2002) 'Melatonin treatment for sleep disorders in children with neuro-developmental disorders: an observational study.' *Developmental Medicine and Child Neurology*, **44**, 339–344.

Russell, D.J., Rosenbaum, P.L., Cadman, D.T., Gowland, C., Hardy, S., Jarvis, S. (1989) 'The Gross Motor Function Measure: a means to evaluate the effects of physical therapy.' *Developmental Medicine and Child Neurology*, **31**, 341–352.

Russell, D.J., Rosenbaum, P.L., Avery, L.M., Lane, M. (2002) *Gross Motor Function Measure (GMFM-66 and GMFM-88) Users Manual. Clinics in Developmental Medicine No. 159.* London: Mac Keith Press.

Rutherford, M.A. (2002) 'Magnetic resonance imaging of injury to the immature brain.' *In:* Squier, W. (Ed.) *Acquired Damage to the Developing Brain.* London: Arnold, pp. 166–192.

Siebes, R., Wijnroks, L., Vermeer, A. (2002) 'Qualitative analysis of the therapeutic intervention programmes for children with cerebral palsy: an update.' *Developmental Medicine and Child Neurology*, **44**, 593–603.

Squier, W. (Ed.) (2002) *Acquired Damage to the Developing Brain—Timing and Causation.* London: Arnold.

Stanley, F.J., Blair, E., Alberman, E. (2000) *Cerebral Palsies: Epidemiology and Causal Pathways. Clinics in Developmental Medicine No. 151.* London: Mac Keith Press.

Steinbok, P., Reiner, A., Beauchamp, R.D., Armstrong, R.W., Cochrane, P.D. (1997) 'A randomized clinical trial to compare selective posterior rhizotomy plus physiotherapy with physiotherapy alone in children with spastic diplegic cerebral palsy.' *Developmental Medicine and Child Neurology*, **39**, 178–184.

Surveillance of Cerebral Palsy in Europe (SCPE) (2002) 'Prevalence and characteristics of children with cerebral palsy in Europe.' *Developmental Medicine and Child Neurology*, **44**, 633–640.

Sutherland, D.H., Olshen, R.A., Biden, E.N., Wyatt, M.P. (1988) *The Development of Mature Walking. Clinics in Developmental Medicine No. 104/105.* London: Mac Keith Press.

Vrbová, G. (1963) 'Changes in the motor reflexes produced by tenotomy.' *Journal of Physiology*, **166**, 241–250.

Wagley, P.F. (1945) 'A study of spasticity and paralysis.' *Bulletin of the Johns Hopkins Hospital*, **71**, 218–273.

Walsh, E.G. (1992) *Muscles Masses and Motion. Clinics in Developmental Medicine No. 125.* London: Mac Keith Press.

Walshe, F.M.R. (1923) 'On certain tonic or postural reflexes in hemiplegia with special reference to the so-called associated movements.' *Brain*, **46**, 281–300.

Wright, F.V., Sheil, E.M., Drake, J.M., Wedge, J.H., Naumann, S. (1998) 'Evaluation of selective dorsal rhizotomy for the reduction of spasticity in cerebral palsy: a randomized controlled trial.' *Developmental Medicine and Child Neurology*, **40**, 239–247.

8
MECHANISMS OF DEFORMITY

H. Kerr Graham

In 1862, William John Little published a monograph entitled *On the Influence of Abnormal Parturition, Difficult Labours, Premature Birth and Asphyxia Neonatorum, on the Mental and Physical Condition of the Child, Especially in Relation to Deformities*. Little had recognized the high incidence of progressive musculoskeletal deformity in the condition known then as "infantile spastic paralysis" and now known as cerebral palsy (CP). Little had a talipes equinovarus, which was successfully treated surgically by a percutaneous tenotomy of the tendo Achillis (Rang 1966). Tenotomy had only just begun to be used in Europe, and following his own experience Little introduced the procedure to England, where it was soon applied to the management of spastic contractures (Green 1975). Orthopaedics is by literal translation 'straight children', and it is appropriate that the first orthopaedic operation was devised for the correction of the most common deformity seen in children with CP, equinus deformity. The connection that Little made between birth trauma and the development of deformities has been overlooked to a remarkable degree in subsequent definitions of CP. Most definitions emphasize the static nature of the cerebral lesion and the variability of the movement disorder. This is undoubtedly helpful in relation to accurate diagnosis but is lacking in relation to the clinical course of the condition and the establishment of management priorities. Furthermore, emphasizing the non-progressive nature of the brain lesion seems to engender a degree of complacency in many clinicians. If the brain lesion is non-progressive, why should the clinical manifestations of the motor disorder be progressive? The development of a painful dislocation of the hip in later childhood may come as an unwelcome surprise to both parents and clinicians. Little clue as to what to expect during childhood is offered by the terms 'static encephalopathy' and 'non-progressive brain lesion'. For these reasons the definition of CP that orthopaedic surgeons find useful emphasizes three key features: (1) CP is a disorder of movement and posture (2) caused by a non-progressive lesion in the immature brain, which amongst other sequelae (3) results in progressive musculoskeletal pathology in the majority of children (Graham 2002).

The brain lesion

Given that CP is the result of a brain lesion or injury and that any or all parts of the brain may be involved, it is not surprising that the clinical manifestations can be so variable and that there are many associated impairments. CP is therefore a useful administrative term, not a precise clinical or pathological diagnosis. The areas of the brain that control movement and posture are the motor cortex, the basal ganglia and the cerebellum. Pure motor disorders resulting from a focal lesion in these three areas would be spastic, dyskinetic and ataxic,

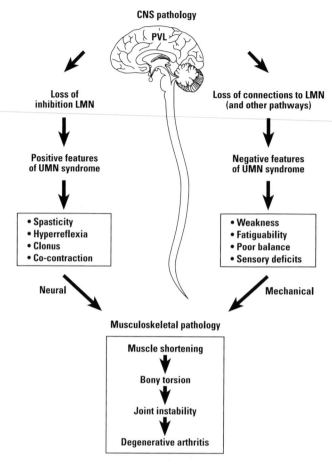

Fig. 8.1. Postulated mechanisms responsible for progressive neuromusculoskeletal pathology in children with cerebral palsy. (Reproduced by permission from Graham and Selber 2003.)

The interaction of the positive and negative features of the upper motor neuron syndrome result in a combination of both neurological and mechanical changes in muscle contributing to fixed contractures, bony torsion and joint instability, which may ultimately lead to premature degenerative arthritis.

respectively. However, focal lesions and pure motor disorders are uncommon. The majority of children have mixed lesions and mixed motor disorders. Recognition of clinical syndromes remains more important than brain imaging in establishing prognosis in the cerebral palsies. Impairments associated with the motor disorder include deficits in cognition, vision, hearing, language and behaviour. Epilepsy, poor nutrition, respiratory disease and dental disease are common medical comorbidities and these may impact on the management of the motor disorder and on the prevention and management of deformities. Imaging modalities, including ultrasound, computed tomography and magnetic resonance imaging, are adding greatly to our understanding of the variability of the brain lesions, which may result in a CP syndrome.

The limb pathology

The spastic and mixed movement disorders account for between 80% and 90% of children with cerebral palsies in current CP registers (Stanley *et al*. 2000). The spastic motor disorders are also associated with the most common disorders of posture, gait and limb deformities and will be the focus of this chapter. The pathology of spasticity cannot be separated from the pathology of the upper motor neuron syndrome (Fig. 8.1). The child with diplegia who toe-walks because of calf spasticity may also be unable to voluntarily control the dorsiflexors of the ankle during gait. No matter how effective management of the calf spasticity is, gait may remain impaired because toe clearance cannot be achieved during the swing phase. Indeed there is virtually always an effective solution to calf spasticity/stiffness/shortening, but inability to control the ankle dorsiflexors during swing phase may mean life-long dependence on an orthosis.

Spasticity is but one feature of the upper motor neuron syndrome. Although clinicians tend to concentrate on its positive features (spasticity, clonus, hyperreflexia, co-contraction), it is the negative features (weakness, loss of selective motor control, sensory impairment) that ultimately may limit function and determine prognosis. Only recently has the importance of weakness in CP been given appropriate recognition (Wiley and Damiano 1998). Muscle strength in children with CP can be measured, and there is some evidence to support the benefits of strengthening programmes (Damiano and Abel 1998, Dodd *et al*. 2002).

Spasticity can be defined as a velocity-dependent resistance to passive movement of a joint and its associated musculature. However, patients do not complain about spasticity, being more likely to be aware of stiffness and deformity. Stiffness is a useful term because it is widely understood by both clinicians and patients. It is also useful in terms of describing limb pathology in patients with spasticity. Although spasticity may be an early problem in the child with CP, true muscle shortening or contracture also appears at an early stage, and the majority of children will have a mixture of spasticity and contracture, the proportions varying with time.

At birth, children with CP do not have contractures, dislocated hips or scoliosis. These common deformities are acquired during childhood. Some years ago, we described musculo-skeletal growth in children with CP as a race between the growth of muscles and the growth of long bones, governed by a biological clock (Boyd and Graham 1997). In this race, the pacemakers are the physes of the long bones, and the muscle–tendon units are doomed to second place. The prerequisite for normal muscle growth is frequent stretching of relaxed muscle. In children with CP the muscles do not readily relax due to spasticity, and they are infrequently stretched because of reduced activity. Activity levels are probably more governed by weakness, impaired balance and poor selective motor control than by spasticity and deformity. Spasticity plus reduced activity leads to failure of longitudinal muscle growth, contractures and fixed deformities (Rang 1990). The speed with which contracture and fixed deformity occurs is very variable and is principally related to the severity of the motor disorder and the rate of growth. The child with mild hemiplegia will develop 1–3 cm of contracture in the gastrocsoleus–Achilles tendon complex between birth and skeletal maturity, usually accompanied by about 2 cm shortening of the tibia on the affected side and 3 cm reduction in the circumference of the calf muscle, compared to the unaffected side.

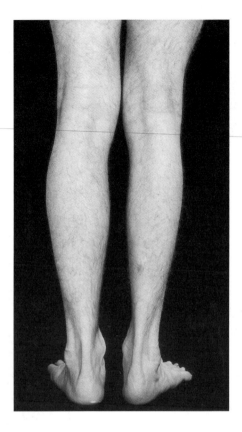

Fig. 8.2. The biological clock in spastic hemiplegia ticks quite slowly, in the majority of children. These are the lower limbs of a young adult with a right hemiplegia at skeletal maturity. Equinus deformity was managed by lengthening of the Achilles tendon at age 8 years. At skeletal maturity there was 2 cm of shortening of the right leg and 3.5 cm of wasting of the right calf.

In hemiplegia the biological clock ticks slowly, speeding up a little during periods of rapid growth, especially the adolescent growth spurt (Fig. 8.2).

Even in hemiplegia, different muscles develop contractures at different rates. The pronator teres is frequently contracted by the age of 3–4 years and may need to be surgically released to regain active supination and to protect the proximal radio-ulnar joint. The long wrist and finger flexors remain spastic rather than contracted until much later in childhood. In severe spastic quadriplegia, the biological clock ticks quickly (Fig. 8.3). The whole cycle from the onset of spasticity in the hip adductors, through fixed contractures and hip subluxation followed by painful hip dislocation, may take only 4–6 years. Understanding the stage of the race helps us to understand the stage of the musculoskeletal pathology. From this understanding, logical management strategies may be developed, whether preventive or reconstructive.

Mechanisms of deformity

The main determinants of deformity in CP are severity of involvement, the type of movement disorder and its topographical distribution. Additional factors are the presence of congenital abnormalities and the modifying influence of management including positioning, physio-

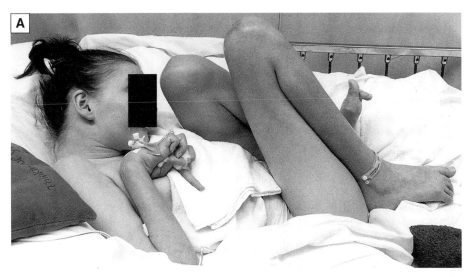

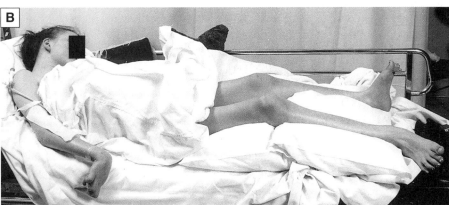

Fig. 8.3. In some children the biological clock may run very quickly, *i.e.* contractures develop very rapidly. (A) This 14-year-old girl presented with full-thickness skin ulceration behind her knees, in her popliteal fossae, over the hamstring tendons and in her elbow flexor creases, over the biceps tendons. This was the result of severe unremitting spastic dystonia that had been present for only two years, as a result of Wilson's disease. She required a combination of spasticity management (intrathecal baclofen pump) and lengthening of the contracted muscle tendon units. Because the contractures were of short duration, it was possible to extend the joints relatively easily. An unexpected bonus was the ability to control foot switches by the left foot for communication (B).

therapy, orthoses and surgery (Brown and Minns 1989). The prognosis for deformity in the child with CP, as for all other important outcomes, is closely related to severity of involvement. It is difficult to prevent progressive deformity in the severely involved child, even with optimal management. Deformities in the minimally involved child are minor and often self-limiting. Spastic movement disorders are more frequently associated with fixed deformity than dystonic, ataxic or hypotonic movement disorders. Topographical involvement in spastic movement disorders points to the likely site for deformity and is in itself another measure of severity. In spastic monoplegia, the deformities are found only in the involved limb and in hemiplegia are restricted to the affected side. In spastic diplegia the principal deformities are in the lower limbs. Spastic quadriplegia is also referred to by some as 'whole body involvement', and the deformities may affect all four limbs and the trunk. The influence of topographical involvement is evident in the incidence of spastic hip displacement, approximately 1% in spastic hemiplegia, 5% in spastic diplegia and more than 50% in spastic quadriplegia (Dobson *et al.* 2002).

The majority of children with CP have no deformities at birth, and few have significant deformities during the first year of life. The majority develop deformities with growth, the exception being a small number of children who are born with congenital abnormalities such as developmental dislocation of the hip.

Natural history

Management during early childhood may influence the incidence, severity and type of deformities seen in children with CP. The natural history of deformity in CP is difficult to define because few populations are untreated. Nevertheless, some observations are possible. Obvious and easily defined deformities such as spinal deformity and spastic hip displacement can be ameliorated or prevented by active management programmes. These major deformities are much more prevalent and much more severe in untreated or poorly treated groups. Contractures seem to be less common and less severe in children who have good access to physiotherapy, orthoses and orthopaedic surgery than in those who do not. In Australia, the contrast between children with CP from rural areas and metropolitan areas can be striking, in terms of the incidence and severity of deformity. Furthermore, in medical systems where access to medical care is unequal, a significant difference in outcome in relation to deformity can be seen in those who have better access compared to those who have less good access. Children involved in therapy systems that prohibit or discourage conventional management have a higher than expected incidence of deformity, especially silent deformities such as hip displacement and spinal deformity. The highest incidence of severe symptomatic deformities is found in institutionalized patients.

The natural history of musculoskeletal deformity and gait deviations is for progressive increase in deformity, even in ambulant children with relatively mild involvement. Two studies, utilizing instrumented gait analysis, have reported progressive deformities and gait deviations in untreated groups of children with CP (Johnson *et al.* 1997, Bell *et al.* 2002). Both studies report decreases in walking speed and increasing flexion contractures and dynamic joint stiffness.

Iatrogenic deformity

The counterpoint to the reduction in deformity as the result of medical intervention is the very real problem of iatrogenic deformity, usually the opposite deformity to the original one (Brown and Minns 1989). In large muscles that demonstrate severe, tonic spasticity, the antagonist group may exhibit reciprocal inhibition. If the spasticity is released by

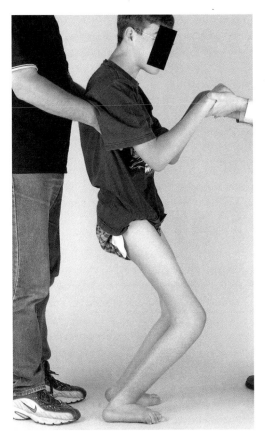

Fig. 8.4. This boy with mild spastic quadriplegia has severe crouch gait and is shown supported in standing by both parents. In early childhood he had bilateral lengthening of the Achilles tendons, which contributed to the severe crouch gait and loss of standing balance and walking ability. Crouch gait may be part of the natural history of both spastic diplegia and spastic quadriplegia, but in many children it is the result of isolated calf-lengthening surgery.

muscle–tendon surgery, reduction in spasticity in the agonist may be accompanied by loss of reciprocal inhibition in the antagonist and the development of the opposite deformity. Crouch gait in spastic diplegia is often caused by surgery for equinus deformity, especially isolated lengthening of the Achilles tendons (Borton *et al*. 2001) (Fig. 8.4). Over-lengthening of the hamstrings can cause recurvatum at the knee, especially if the calf is contracted or spastic. Overly enthusiastic lengthening of the hip adductors can cause abduction contracture of the hip, especially when combined with casting of the hips in excessive abduction for a long period of time. The most common reasons for iatrogenic deformities are the failure to distinguish between dynamic and fixed deformities and the failure to differentiate a primary problem from a secondary, compensatory response (Gage 1991). Primary problems require treatment. When treatment is successful, the coping response will then resolve. Children with hemiplegia and a unilateral equinus deformity will often 'vault' on the unaffected side, to help with clearance. Vaulting may be so persistent that stiffness in the gastrocsoleus in the unaffected side can be detected on examination. After successful unilateral equinus surgery, the vaulting response is no longer required and will resolve.

The limb pathology: general observations

The general sequence in the genesis of deformity is abnormal posture and dynamic deformity, followed by fixed musculo-tendinous contracture. Tonic spasticity and rigidity are more commonly associated with more rapidly progressive deformities than phasic spasticity. The more severely involved the child, the more severe the weakness and loss of selective motor control. Those children who cannot walk are more liable to severe, fixed deformity than those who walk with assistance. The persistence of neonatal postural asymmetry, combined with immobility, may set the scene for severe asymmetric limb deformities in later life, such as 'windswept hips' (Brown and Minns 1989). Those children who walk independently are relatively protected from severe deformity by postural changes, alternating agonist–antagonist muscle activity, better strength and better selective motor control. Growth of the musculoskeletal system is also related to severity. Children with severe spastic quadriplegia frequently have marked global reduction in growth, which is multifactorial in origin. Focal or asymmetric growth restriction is seen with asymmetric neurological involvement, such as in spastic hemiplegia and asymmetric diplegia.

Understanding the progressive nature of the musculoskeletal pathology has been achieved from both animal and clinical studies. In the hereditary spastic mouse, Ziv *et al.* (1984) demonstrated a failure of longitudinal growth of the muscle–tendon unit in relation to bone length and the development of a fixed contracture. However, Cosgrove and Graham (1994) showed that injection of botulinum toxin A into the gastrocnemius muscle of juvenile spastic mice promotes more normal growth and prevents contractures, by reducing spasticity. The addition or subtraction of sarcomeres is an adaptation to enable a muscle to work in its optimal range. It has been shown that splinting of a muscle in a shortened state is associated with a reduction of up to 40% in the number of sarcomeres in series. Conversely, if the joint is splinted in extension, the number of sarcomeres in series can be increased by up to 25% (Tabary *et al.* 1972, Williams and Goldspink 1978). These experiments on muscle adaptation to imposed length changes have profound implications in both the understanding of the origin and prevention of fixed muscle–tendon contractures.

Muscles are not the only soft tissue to be affected in CP, and the periarticular connective tissues are also prone to contracture, probably because of relative immobility rather than changes in muscle length. Children with CP have a global reduction in activity compared to their peers, and individual joints may function through a reduced range because of specific physiological and biomechanical circumstances. Muscle contracture is closely related to length changes, but stiffness in periarticular connective changes is related to movement deprivation (Akeson *et al.* 1987). Again, management implications are clear but difficult to achieve. Prevention of muscle and connective tissue contracture may require maintenance of individual muscle length and a good overall level of activity. This may be feasible in mild diplegia but is probably not feasible for children with severe quadriplegia.

Spastic CP is 'short muscle disease', and muscle shortening can have serious deleterious consequences on the growing skeleton, including bony torsion, joint instability, joint dislocation and degenerative arthritis (Rang 1990). Spastic CP is therefore a static encephalopathy with progressive musculoskeletal deformity (Graham 2002).

In the younger child, deformities are mainly dynamic. In the lower limb, they are

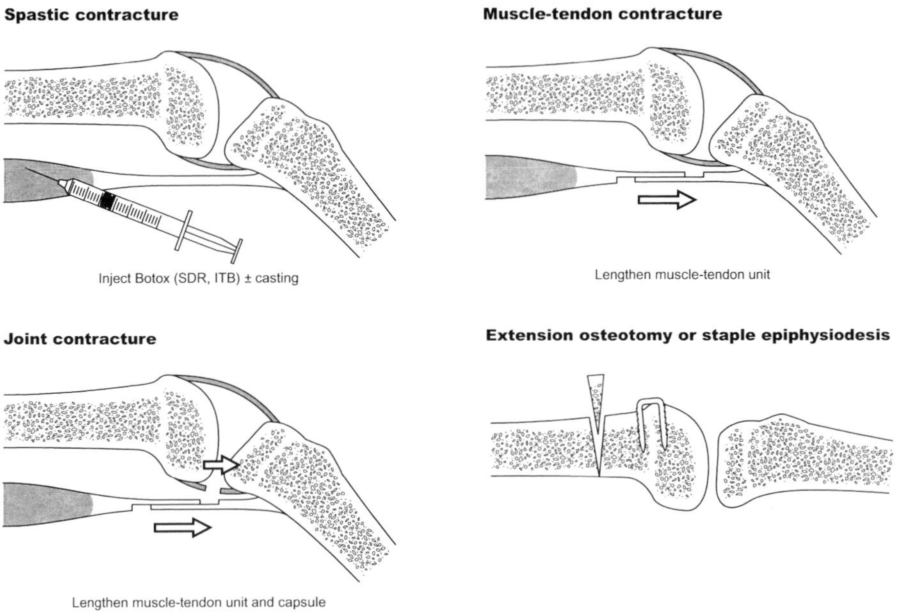

Inject Botox (SDR, ITB) ± casting

Lengthen muscle-tendon unit

Joint contracture

Extension osteotomy or staple epiphysiodesis

Lengthen muscle-tendon unit and capsule

Fig. 8.5. Management of deformities in children with cerebral palsy is directly related to the stage of the musculoskeletal pathology. For a spastic contracture, the options are focal spasticity treatment such as injection of the muscle with botulinum toxin A or, if more generalized spasticity management is required, selective dorsal rhizotomy or intrathecal baclofen. Once a fixed muscle–tendon contracture has developed, surgical lengthening is required. At the stage of joint contracture, lengthening of the muscle–tendon unit and release of the joint capsule is necessary. For neglected deformities, extension osteotomy or stapling of the anterior part of the epiphysis may be required to effect a complete correction.

obvious when the child attempts to walk and are more pronounced if the child is stressed. Dynamic deformities are less pronounced when the child is relaxed or asleep, and by definition disappear completely under anaesthesia. Deformities may remain dynamic in dystonic movement disorders but usually progress to fixed deformity in mixed and spastic movement disorders. Fixed deformities are still present when the child is relaxed under anaesthesia. Musculoskeletal deformities affect soft tissues, bones and joints. Soft-tissue pathology includes muscle contracture and connective tissue changes (Fig. 8.5). Pathology in the long bones includes torsional deformities, angular deformities and growth inhibition. Joint pathology includes capsular contractures, joint instability, subluxation and dislocation, as well as damage to articular cartilage and degenerative arthritis. The harmful effects of immobilization on synovial joints are well known from animal experiments (Salter and Field 1960, Akeson *et al.* 1977). Immobilization in extreme positions is even more harmful. Eccentric loading of synovial joints is damaging to hyaline articular cartilage, which has very limited powers of regeneration—hence the need to prevent the adverse biomechanical environment in childhood that may lead to premature degenerative arthritis in early adult life. The most serious musculoskeletal problem faced by young adults with CP is painful,

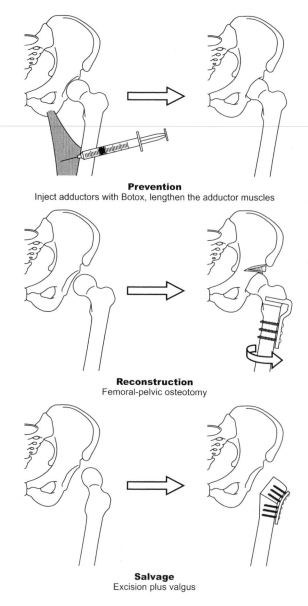

Prevention
Inject adductors with Botox, lengthen the adductor muscles

Reconstruction
Femoral-pelvic osteotomy

Salvage
Excision plus valgus

Fig. 8.6. Management of spastic hip displacement is related to the stage of the musculoskeletal pathology. In the very early stages of hip displacement, preventive treatment can be considered such as injecting the adductors of the hip with botulinum toxin A or lengthening of the adductor muscles for fixed contracture. This is effective in the majority of younger children. If the hip is severely displaced, reconstructive surgery is required, usually a combination of femoral and pelvic osteotomy. However, if the femoral head is severely damaged in a neglected dislocation, reconstruction of the hip may be impossible and the only remaining option is some form of salvage surgery. Excision of the damaged femoral head combined with a valgus femoral osteotomy may reduce pain but is a poor substitute for a normal hip joint.

premature, degenerative arthritis with approximately 20% experiencing pain on a daily basis (Andersson and Mattsson 2001). Management is difficult and unsatisfactory. Prevention is a much better strategy and must commence in childhood by the early, effective management of deformities (Fig. 8.6).

The concept of decompensation

Decompensation is a critical concept in understanding musculoskeletal pathology and management of fixed deformity in CP. The body will adapt advantageously to compensate for shortcomings, but there comes a point where the body's efforts to adapt to the situation set up secondary pathologies and compensation becomes disadvantageous. We use the term to define a threshold that exists between muscle pathology and joint pathology in the child with CP. The muscle pathology consists of spasticity, stiffness and contracture of muscle–tendon units and supporting connective tissues, to varying degrees. The joint pathology is contracture of joint capsule and collateral ligaments followed by changes in joint shape, loss of articular cartilage, intra-articular deformity, instability and degenerative arthritis. The management of the muscle pathology is spasticity management and contracture surgery. The prognosis for improving or maintaining function is good, and complications following intervention are infrequent. In the phase of decompensated musculoskeletal pathology, management is dominated by salvage surgery, maintaining function is very difficult, and surgical complication rates are very high.

In the child with spastic diplegia, the onset of fixed flexion deformity at the knee is the key clinical sign of moving into the phase of decompensation. No matter how high the popliteal angle, flexed knee gait is easily corrected by lengthening of the hamstrings in the absence of fixed flexion deformity of the joint. Once fixed flexion deformity at the knee exceeds about 20°, complete correction of flexed knee gait is difficult, and the incidence of common peroneal nerve palsy after hamstring lengthening increases four-fold.

In spastic hip displacement, prior to decompensation, the hip adductors are spastic and may be contracted but the femoral head is round, it may be subluxated but not dislocated, and secondary acetabular dysplasia is absent or present to a minor degree. Soft-tissue surgery is sufficient to prevent hip dislocation in 70% of hips prior to decompensation, and reconstructive surgery (femoral or pelvic osteotomy) will ensure a good result in the remainder (Miller *et al.* 1995) (Figs. 8.7, 8.8) After decompensation, reconstructive surgery is difficult, the results are indifferent, and many hips have to be managed by salvage surgery. At the most extreme, this means excising the irreparably damaged femoral head (Fig. 8.9).

Decompensation is less frequent in spastic hemiplegia but may occur in both the upper and lower limb. In spastic equinus prior to decompensation, the equinus contracture is easily managed by lengthening of the gastrocsoleus and the provision of an ankle–foot orthosis. After decompensation, contractures of the ankle and subtalar joint capsules may occur and secondary bony deformities of the mid-foot and forefoot may occur. At this stage bony surgery for mid-foot breaching and operations for painful bunions may be required (Goldstein and Harper 2001). In the hemiplegic upper limb, pronation deformity can be managed by pronator teres re-routing. However, decompensation may be associated with

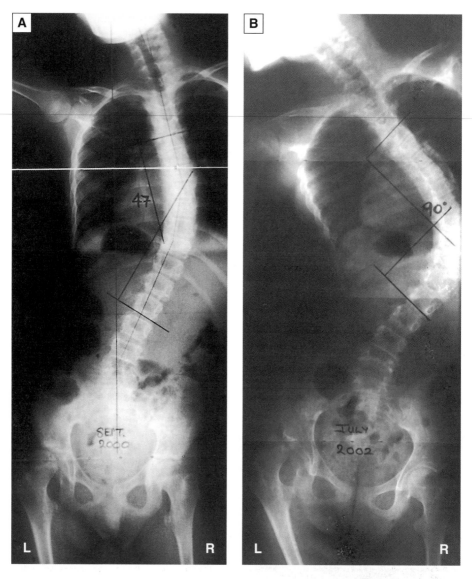

Fig. 8.7A. Posteroanterior X-ray of the spine, pelvis and hips of a 12-year-old girl with mild spastic quadriplegia. She has a thoracolumbar scoliosis measuring 47°, convex to the right, mild pelvic obliquity and a subluxed left hip. Her surgeon recommended reconstructive surgery for the left hip and close monitoring of the scoliosis with a view to early surgical correction. The family chose to embark on a course of chiropractic treatment and did not attend for further examination or X-ray for 22 months.

B. Twenty-two months later, the scoliosis had progressed to 90°, and the left hip had dislocated and was painful. At this stage the hip was severely damaged and subsequently required excision. It was too late for reconstructive surgery. The scoliosis now requires two-stage spinal surgery with greatly increased risk of morbidity and mortality. This is an example of decompensation. During the adolescent growth spurt, deformities can progress very rapidly and the option for reconstructive surgery may be missed within a single year. Close follow-up is particularly important during periods of rapid growth.

116

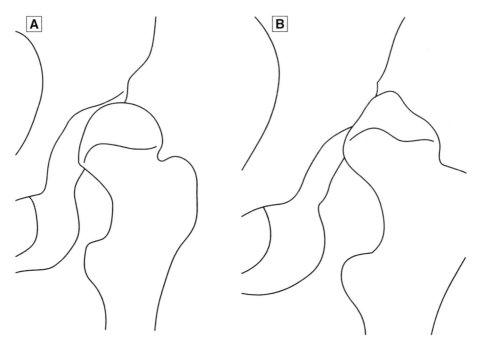

Fig. 8.8. Tracings (from anteroposterior radiographs) of the shape of the left femoral head, which is difficult to see in the X-rays in Figure 8.7. (A) At first presentation the femoral head is round, and although it is subluxed, reconstructive surgery would have been successful. (B) Twenty-two months later the femoral head is deformed and reconstructive surgery is no longer possible.

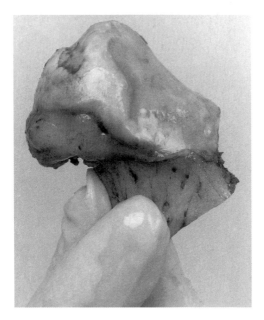

Fig. 8.9. This is the femoral head that was surgically removed from the patient described in Figures 8.7 and 8.8. Instead of the normal spherical shape, covered with glistening hyaline articular cartilage, the femoral head has become triangular and almost all of the articular cartilage has been eroded. Once the femoral head is damaged by eccentric pressure on the edge of the acetabulum and against the spastic hip abductors, reconstructive surgery is no longer feasible and this type of salvage surgery is the only remaining option.

contracture of the interosseous membrane and radial head dislocation, which precludes a successful outcome.

The limb pathology: topograhical survey

SPASTIC HEMIPLEGIA

The majority of children with spastic hemiplegia develop flexion/pronation deformities in the upper limb and equinus in the lower limb.

The upper-limb deformities typically include internal rotation and adduction at the shoulder, and this may progress in a small minority of patients to anterior migration of the humeral head or dislocation of the gleno-humeral joint. The pectoralis major and the subscapularis are usually the main deforming forces. Severe adduction/internal rotation contracture of the gleno-humeral joint may rarely be associated with premature, rapidly progressive degenerative arthritis in young adults, with spastic hemiplegia.

At the elbow, flexion deformity is very common, initially dynamic, progressing to a fixed deformity with variable degrees of joint contracture. In the forearm, pronation deformities are ubiquitous and are the result of spastic pronators (pronator teres and pronator quadratus) with weak or paralysed supinators. Loss of active supination results in a contracture in the interosseous membrane and may predispose to subluxation or dislocation of the radial head. Flexion deformities of the wrist and fingers are the most common deformities in the upper limb, because the spastic flexors overpower the weaker extensors. Wrist flexion deformity is usually accompanied by ulnar deviation because the ulnar deviators are more powerful than the radial deviators.

The 'thumb-in-palm' deformity is very common and is associated with significant functional impairment. The posture is one of adduction or adduction and flexion, the result of spasticity in the adductor pollicis, the flexor pollicis brevis and the first dorsal interosseous. In long-standing cases secondary pathology may develop in the metacarpophalangeal joint of the thumb.

As with all deformities, there is a postural–dynamic phase with gradual development of fixed contracture of the muscle–tendon units. Eventually, this leads to the phase of decompensation, which may include subluxation/dislocation of the gleno-humeral joint, fixed elbow contracture, fixed pronation/flexion in the forearm and wrist, and dislocation of the radial head. Different muscles develop fixed contractures at different speeds. The pronator teres is invariably the first muscle in the hemiplegic upper limb to develop a contracture (Boyd and Graham 1997). This is not because it is more spastic than other muscles but because it is never stretched by antagonist action. Loss of active supination is present to some degree in all children with hemiplegia. Prevention of pronation contracture is simple in principle but very difficult in practice. The pronator teres must be stretched out to its maximum length by the parent or therapist because the child is unable to do this. Contractures of the wrist and finger flexors remain dynamic for many years, and this has important implications for management. The combination of pronator teres lengthening (or re-routing) combined with intramuscular injections of botulinum toxin A to the wrist and finger flexors is appropriate for many children (Graham 2001).

Muscle imbalance is important in the genesis of upper-limb deformities. The stronger flexors and pronators tend to overcome the less powerful extensors and supinators. This is the reason why deformities are so stereotyped in the hemiplegic upper limb and in spastic CP in general.

In the lower limb, spasticity and contractures are more pronounced distally than proximally. Equinus is very common, and hip involvement is unusual. Tonic spasticity of the gastrocsoleus is usually associated with reciprocal inhibition of the dorsiflexors of the ankle. However, equinus deformity is not the result of imbalance between the plantarflexors and dorsiflexors of the ankle but of that between the plantarflexors and the ground reaction force (Silver *et al.* 1985). The plantarflexors are more than six times as strong as the dorsiflexors and they are active at different times in the gait cycle. Management is therefore focused not on re-establishing balance between these muscle groups but on ensuring appropriate functional length in the gastrocsoleus during second rocker, while preserving strength for push-off during third rocker. Effective management of calf spasticity or contracture is often associated with improved function in the ankle dorsiflexors, occasionally to the point of producing a calcaneus deformity. In comparison with the upper limb, the progression from spastic contracture to fixed contracture is much more rapid. This has important management implications. Spasticity management in the lower limb is only effective in younger children; injections of botulinum toxin A are useful from age 2 to 6 years (Cosgrove *et al.* 1994). Equinus in most children over the age of 6 years requires muscle–tendon lengthening. Equinovarus and equinovalgus deformities are also common and require tendon transfer procedures and bony stabilization operations respectively. The Winters and Gage classification of gait in spastic hemiplegia is very helpful in the recognition of the spastic motor patterns and in the subsequent development of patterns of fixed deformity (Winters *et al.* 1987) (Fig. 8.10).

In Group I hemiplegia there is a foot drop in swing phase but there are no fixed deformities. The drop foot is the result of loss of selective motor control, a negative feature of the upper motor neuron syndrome. As there is no contracture or joint deformity, management is by the prescription of a leaf-spring or hinged ankle–foot orthosis (AFO). Contracture surgery and deformity correction are not required.

In Group II hemiplegia there is a fixed equinus contracture at the ankle with no proximal contractures. This is by far the most common type. Management requires lengthening of the gastrocsoleus by injection of botulinum toxin A in the dynamic phase or by lengthening of the tendo Achillis in the fixed contracture phase, and the provision of a hinged AFO.

In Group III hemiplegia, in addition to equinus at the ankle there is involvement at the knee, with co-contraction of the hamstrings and quadriceps. In addition to lengthening of the gastrocsoleus, the hamstrings may require lengthening and the rectus femoris may need to be transferred to semitendinosus, for stiff-knee gait.

In Group IV hemiplegia, there is involvement at the ankle, knee and hip levels, with equinus contracture at the ankle, co-contraction at the knee and flexion–adduction and internal rotation at the hip. Management is as for group III, with the addition of lengthening of the hip adductors and flexors, and when necessary femoral derotation osteotomy.

In spastic hemiplegia, there is usually asymmetric growth of the limbs including diminished longitudinal growth, diminished circumferential growth, and a reduction in glove size

119

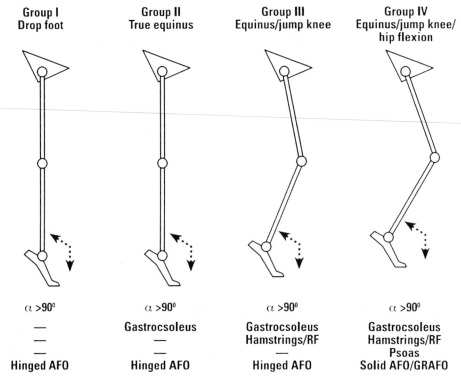

Group I Drop foot	Group II True equinus	Group III Equinus/jump knee	Group IV Equinus/jump knee/ hip flexion
α >90⁰	α >90⁰	α >90⁰	α >90⁰
—	Gastrocsoleus	Gastrocsoleus	Gastrocsoleus
—	—	Hamstrings/RF	Hamstrings/RF
—	—	—	Psoas
Hinged AFO	Hinged AFO	Hinged AFO	Solid AFO/GRAFO

Fig. 8.10. The classification of gait patterns in spastic hemiplegia by Winters *et al.* (1987) is a useful guide to management.

in the upper limb and shoe size in the lower limb. The difference in lower-limb length at maturity averages 2.5cm, which is enough to affect gait in some individuals and to require limb equalization surgery, by epiphysiodesis, in a minority (Graham and Fixsen 1988) (see Fig. 8.2).

SPASTIC DIPLEGIA

In spastic diplegia there is spasticity, followed by contracture at all three anatomical/levels in the lower limbs: hip, knee and ankle–foot (Fig. 8.11). At the hip there is flexion/adduction/ internal rotation; at the knee, flexed–stiff knee gait; and at the ankle, equinus, usually accompanied by valgus and less commonly varus. Spastic hip displacement is uncommon, occurring in about 5% of children, usually assisted ambulators, with independent ambulators relatively protected. Pelvic obliquity and scoliosis are relatively rare and usually mild. Spasticity and contracture have their principal effects on the large lower-limb muscle groups, which act mainly in the sagittal plane and which cross two joints. These include the psoas, the hamstrings, the rectus femoris and the gastrocnemius. The iliacus, the vasti and the soleus cross only one joint and usually are not affected (Bache *et al.* 2003).

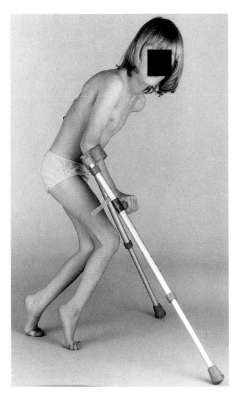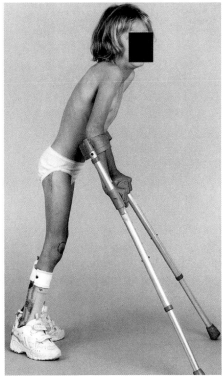

Fig. 8.11. The classic three-level contractures in severe spastic diplegia resulting in 'jump gait'. There are fixed contractures of the hip flexors, the hamstrings and the gastrocsoleus. This was managed by multilevel surgery including lengthening of the iliopsoas at the brim of the pelvis, fractional lengthening of the medial hamstrings, and lengthening of the gastrocnemius aponeurosis. The sagittal alignment is seen postoperatively, and the child is now able to wear ankle–foot orthoses comfortably.

Spasticity, contractures and weakness are manifested in a number of characteristic gait patterns, which have been described by different terms by a succession of authors. Based on a combination of pattern recognition and kinematic analysis, we have devised a simple four-group classification: equinus gait, jump gait, apparent equinus and crouch gait (Rodda and Graham 2001) (Fig. 8.12) Patterns characterized by flexion at the hip and knee are much more common than in spastic hemiplegia because of the insidious effects of bilateral lower limb weakness and lever arm disease.

Group I: true equinus. In true equinus, the ankle is in equinus and the knee and hip are in extension. Most younger children with spastic diplegia walk in a pattern of true equinus and can be managed by intramuscular injection of botulinum toxin A, combined with AFOs. However, by the time fixed contractures of the gastrocsoleus have developed, there are usually occult contractures of the hamstrings and hip flexors that may require correction. Posterior leaf-spring or articulated AFOs are usually indicated.

121

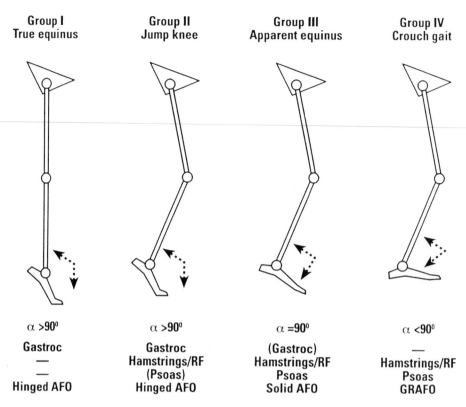

Group I True equinus	Group II Jump knee	Group III Apparent equinus	Group IV Crouch gait
α >90⁰	α >90⁰	α =90⁰	α <90⁰
Gastroc	Gastroc	(Gastroc)	—
—	Hamstrings/RF	Hamstrings/RF	Hamstrings/RF
—	(Psoas)	Psoas	Psoas
Hinged AFO	Hinged AFO	Solid AFO	GRAFO

Fig. 8.12. The classification of sagittal gait patterns by Rodda and Graham (2001) is a template for understanding gait patterns, musculoskeletal pathology and management.

Group II: jump gait. Jump gait is characterized by spasticity, followed by contracture at all three anatomic levels, pelvis–hip, knee and ankle–foot. At initial contact, the hip and knee are excessively flexed and the ankle is in plantarflexion or equinus. During stance, both the hip and the knee extend and the centre of gravity moves upwards to an excessive degree as if the child were jumping. Posterior leaf spring or articulated AFOs may be indicated.

Group III: apparent equinus. In apparent equinus, the child walks on their toes, only because of excessive flexion at the knee and hip. However, the equinus is apparent and not real. Proximal muscle–tendon recessions are called for, not botulinum toxin injections or lengthening of the calf muscle. The increased support of solid AFOs is also usually required.

Group IV: crouch gait. In crouch gait the ankle is in calcaneus and the knees and hips are very flexed. Lengthening of the contracted hamstrings and psoas are required, with the provision of a ground-reaction AFO and correction of bony deformities.

In addition to contractures of muscle–tendon units, torsional deformities and deformation of joints are common in diplegia. The typical torsional deformities are medial femoral

122

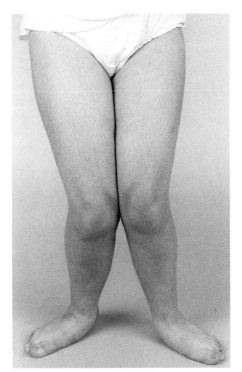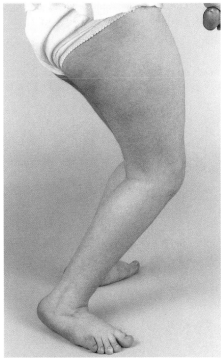

Fig. 8.13. Torsional deformities of the femur and tibia, in combination with deformities of the foot, are collectively referred to as 'lever arm disease'. This girl has a combination of medial femoral torsion, lateral tibial torsion, valgus pronated feet and deformities of the forefeet. The malalignment of the skeletal levers further impairs the effectiveness of muscles and frequently results in 'crouch gait'. [Reproduced by permission from Rodda and Graham (2001).]

torsion and lateral tibial torsion. Medial femoral torsion is the result of failure of fetal femoral alignment to remodel. External tibial torsion is acquired as the result of disordered biomechanics of walking. The common joint deformities are midfoot breaching with valgus hindfoot and abductus of the forefoot. Hallux valgus and flexion deformities of the lesser toes are also common. The bony pathology is sometimes referred to collectively as 'lever arm disease'. The bones and joints are the levers on which the motors, the muscles, work. If a bony lever is maldirected (bony torsion) or unstable (joint subluxation), the efficiency of the muscle in generating an effective moment is greatly reduced. Hence, the soft-tissue pathology (muscle contractures) and the bony pathology (lever arm disease) interact to impair the function of individual joints or limb segments, as well as causing overall impairment of gait (Gage 1991) (Fig. 8.13).

SPASTIC QUADRIPLEGIA, "WHOLE BODY INVOLVEMENT"
In spastic quadriplegia the motor disorder is much more severe, with a combination of severe weakness, loss of selective motor control, retention of primitive reflexes and total

movement patterns, and severe generalized spasticity. These children are unable to walk, and many are completely dependent for all aspects of their care. The deforming forces include spasticity, muscle imbalance, abnormal posturing and the effects of gravity.

The limb deformities are often severe, asymmetric and accompanied by trunk deformities including pelvic obliquity and spinal deformity. Limb deformities are common and often severe but may be overshadowed by the unwelcome triad of unilateral hip dislocation, pelvic obliquity and scoliosis (see Fig. 8.7). The interrelationship of these three deformities may be causal and temporally related but not always easy to elucidate. Many children follow a path characterized by slow and asymmetric hip subluxation with unilateral hip dislocation, followed by the rapid development of pelvic obliquity (high on the side of the dislocation) and scoliosis, convex towards the side of the dislocated hip.

Windswept hip deformity is common and difficult to manage (Letts *et al.* 1984) (Figs. 8.14, 8.15). One hip is flexed, adducted and internally rotated and the contralateral hip is abducted and externally rotated and may appear to be flexed but is usually extended. The adducted hip is usually subluxated or dislocated and the abducted hip is hyper-enlocated (Fig. 8.15). A careful examination awake, under anaesthesia, supplemented by radiographs is required before deciding which are the deforming forces and what should be done to manage deformity and pain. Although it has been suggested that neonatal asymmetry may be a pre-disposing cause of windswept deformity, we consider the deformity to be multifactorial (Brown and Minns 1989). Abduction contracture of the hip is frequently a much more severe deforming force than adduction deformity and much more difficult to manage. Abduction deformity may be a primary deformity or an iatrogenic deformity secondary to adductor release surgery. Factors that increase the risk of abduction deformity after adductor surgery are excessively radical muscle releases, obturator neurectomy, and excessive abduction in casts after surgery, for long periods of time. Abduction deformity is so difficult to manage that some surgeons have advised against obturator neurectomy in all children. In the present author's opinion, however, anterior branch obturator neurectomy is valuable in severe spastic hip disease, although great care must be taken to maintain symmetry after surgery and to avoid the other risk factors for abduction contracture. I therefore use abduction casts in 20–30° of abduction for each hip, for a total of 40–60°. The period of casting is limited to three weeks.

Spinal deformities are common and may be postural or fixed. Postural deformities are usually exaggeration of normal physiological postures, kyphosis in the dorsal spine and lordosis in the lumbar spine. They are caused by weakness and muscle imbalance. Mild to moderate flexible spinal deformities in the younger child should be managed by careful observation, custom seating and occasionally bracing. Bracing is rarely tolerated and therefore usually ineffective in children with severe spastic quadriplegia. Careful positioning and optimal seating are more effective than a spinal orthosis, which is rarely worn because of poor tolerance. Prevention of spinal deformity is inextricably linked to prevention of pelvic obliquity and prevention of fixed hip deformity and hip dislocation. Spastic hip disease is so prevalent in spastic quadriplegia that the majority of children will require surgical intervention by age 10 years (Scrutton *et al.* 2001). In the early stages, spastic hip displacement is silent and not always easy to detect by clinical examination (Fig. 8.16). Hip surveillance

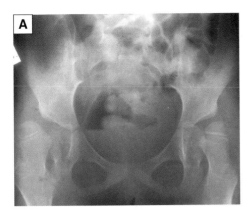
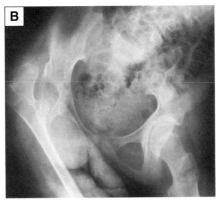

Fig. 8.14A. Bilateral hip subluxation in an 8-year-old child with spastic quadriplegia. Note that the pelvis is level but the hip displacement is asymmetric. The migration percentage on the right is 70% and on the left it is 50%. At this stage the femoral heads are round and both hips could be managed by reconstructive surgery with a good outcome expected.

B. Six years later, the right hip has dislocated, the pelvis has become very oblique and severe scoliosis has developed. The right hip is painful, the patient has great difficulty sitting, and there is no satisfactory surgical management for these 'windswept hips'.

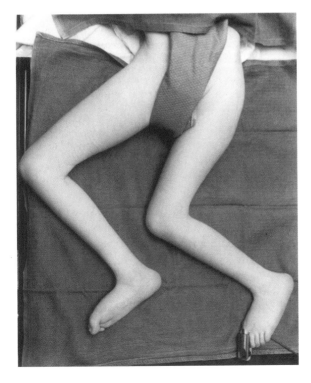

Fig. 8.15. The windswept deformity. The right hip is abducted and externally rotated; the left hip is adducted and internally rotated. The right hip is hyper-enlocated and the left hip has a painful dislocation. Such severe deformities can usually be prevented by close surveillance and by appropriate early intervention.

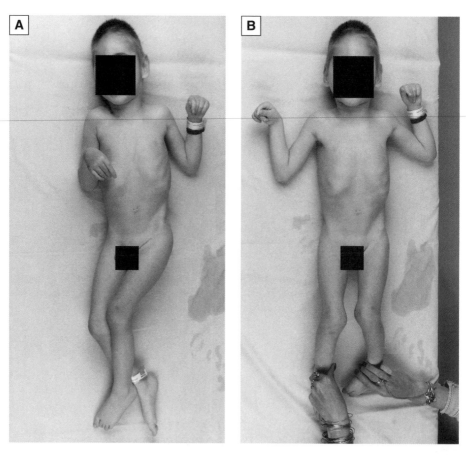

Fig. 8.16A. Hip displacement is silent in younger children with cerebral palsy and can be detected only by a combination of clinical and radiological examination. In this 3-year-old boy with spastic quadriplegia there is a 'scissoring posture' and apparent shortening of the left lower limb.

B. This is the maximum range of abduction possible, and on radiological examination both hips were found to be significantly displaced. Because of the high risk of silent hip displacement, all children with spastic quadriplegia should have regular clinical and radiological examination of their hips from the age of 30 months.

is therefore recommended either by the individual child's physiotherapist, paediatrician, or surgeon or by linking into local hip surveillance programmes, if available (Scrutton and Baird 1997, Dobson *et al.* 2002). Systematic screening of all children with spastic quadriplegia, linked to a local CP register, offers the best opportunity of eliminating the scourge of late spastic hip disease. All children should have their first hip radiograph by age 30 months and this should be repeated every 6–12 months according to clinical and radiographic signs of progression (Scrutton and Baird 1997, Dobson *et al.* 2002).

The development of a unilateral hip dislocation often heralds the development of rapidly progressive scoliosis, with a wide variety of curve patterns recorded. The spinal deformities are often flexible in the early stages, as demonstrated on bending films, but may rapidly become fixed. Deformities, which start in early childhood, are liable to become more severe, more rigid and result in greater cardiorespiratory compromise than those that develop in late childhood. Spinal deformities in CP have a greater risk of curve progression after skeletal maturity than non-neuromuscular spinal deformities.

Before decompensation, when the curves are relatively flexible, a long posterior instrumented spinal fusion to the pelvis may be adequate. Single-stage posterior surgery is relatively well tolerated by the patient and has a good success rate. After decompensation, the spinal deformities may become so fixed that combined anterior and posterior surgery, or staged operations, may be required. These carry greatly increased risk of morbidity and mortality, with decreased deformity correction (Miller *et al.* 1995).

Limb deformities in spastic quadriplegia are similar to those seen in spastic hemiplegia and spastic diplegia but are often more severe and more asymmetric. Many children with quadriplegia have generalized osteopenia, which is multifactorial in origin. Contributing factors are diminished weight bearing, poor nutrition, and medications for the control of epilepsy which have an anti-vitamin D effect. The result is a high incidence of insufficiency fractures, especially after postoperative immobilization (Bischof *et al.* 2002).

In the upper limb, preservation of limited hand function may enable the child to use communication devices and wheelchair controls. Combinations of focal spasticity management, occupational therapy, splinting and soft-tissue surgery may help optimize upper-limb function. The smallest gain in function may have an enormous impact on independence.

Mild flexion deformities at the hips and knees have little impact on the ability to stand for transfers, but painful, deformed feet are a major hindrance. Prevention of rapidly progressive deformity can usually be achieved in younger children by bracing, casting and focal spasticity management. A careful combination of soft-tissue surgery and bony stabilization surgery is usually required to achieve and maintain comfortable, plantigrade feet in the older child.

Conclusion

Cerebral palsy is a static encephalopathy that is associated with progressive musculoskeletal pathology and fixed deformity in the majority of children. Severe physical deformities, which impair self-esteem, function and quality of life, should not be considered to be acceptable in children with CP. Deformities can be prevented or ameliorated by a well-planned and carefully coordinated plan of management. This will be addressed in the following chapter.

REFERENCES

Akeson, W.H., Amiel, D., Mechanic, G.L., Woo, S.L., Harwood, F.L., Hamer, M.L. (1977). 'Collagen cross-linking alterations in joint contractures: changes in the reducible cross-links in periarticular connective tissue collagen after nine weeks of immobilization.' *Connective Tissue Research*, **5**, 15–19.

Akeson, W.H., Amiel, D., Abel, M.F., Garfin, S.R., Woo, S.L. (1987) 'Effects of immobilization on joints.' *Clinical Orthopaedics and Related Research*, **219**, 28–37.

Andersson, C., Mattsson, E. (2001) 'Adults with cerebral palsy: a survey describing problems, needs, and resources, with special emphasis on locomotion.' *Developmental Medicine and Child Neurology*, **43**, 76–82.

Bache, C.E., Selber, P., Graham, H.K. (2003) 'The management of spastic diplegia.' *Current Orthopaedics*, **17**, 88–104.

Bell, K.J., Ounpuu, S., DeLuca, P.A., Romness, M.J. (2002) 'Natural progression of gait in children with cerebral palsy.' *Journal of Pediatric Orthopedics*, **22**, 677–682.

Bischof, F., Basu, D., Pettifor, J.M. (2002) 'Pathological long-bone fractures in residents with cerebral palsy in a long-term care facility in South Africa.' *Developmental Medicine and Child Neurology*, **44**, 119–122.

Borton, D.C., Walker, K., Pirpiris, M., Nattrass, G.R., Graham, H.K. (2001) 'Isolated calf lengthening in cerebral palsy. Outcome analysis of risk factors.' *Journal of Bone and Joint Surgery, British Volume*, **83**, 364–370.

Boyd, R.N., Graham, H.K. (1997) 'Botulinum toxin A in the management of children with cerebral palsy: indications and outcome.' *European Journal of Neurology*, **4** (Suppl. 2), S15–S22.

Brown, J.K., Minns, R.A. (1989) 'Mechanisms of deformity in children with cerebral palsy.' *Seminars in Orthopaedics*, **14**, 236–255.

Cosgrove, A.P., Graham, H.K. (1994) 'Botulinum toxin A prevents the development of contractures in the hereditary spastic mouse.' *Developmental Medicine and Child Neurology*, **36**, 379–385.

Cosgrove, A.P., Corry, I.S., Graham, H.K. (1994) 'Botulinum toxin in the management of the lower limb in cerebral palsy.' *Developmental Medicine and Child Neurology*, **36**, 386–396.

Damiano, D.L., Abel, M.F. (1998) 'Functional outcomes of strength training in spastic cerebral palsy.' *Archives of Physical Medicine and Rehabilitation*, **79**, 119–125.

Dobson, F., Boyd, R.N., Parrott, J., Nattrass, G.R., Graham, H.K. (2002) 'Hip surveillance in children with cerebral palsy.' *Journal of Bone and Joint Surgery, British Volume*, **84**, 720–726.

Dodd, K.J., Taylor, N.F., Damiano, D.L. (2002) 'A systematic review of the effectiveness of strength-training programs for people with cerebral palsy.' *Archives of Physical Medicine and Rehabilitation*, **83**, 1157–1164.

Gage, J.R. (1991) *Gait Analysis in Cerebral Palsy. Clinics in Developmental Medicine No. 121.* London: Mac Keith Press.

Goldstein, M., Harper, D.C. (2001) 'Management of cerebral palsy: equinus gait.' *Developmental Medicine and Child Neurology*, **43**, 563–569.

Graham, H.K. (2001) 'Botulinum toxin type A management of spasticity in the context of orthopaedic surgery for children with spastic cerebral palsy.' *European Journal of Neurology*, **8** (Suppl. 5), 30–39.

Graham, H.K. (2002) 'Painful hip dislocation in cerebral palsy.' *Lancet*, **359**, 907–908.

Graham, H.K., Fixsen, J.A. (1988) 'Lengthening of the calcaneal tendon in spastic hemiplegia by the White slide technique. A long-term review.' *Journal of Bone and Joint Surgery, British Volume*, **70**, 472–475.

Graham, H.K., Selber, P. (2003) 'Musculoskeletal aspects of cerebral palsy.' *Journal of Bone and Joint Surgery, British Volume*, **85**, 157–166.

Green, W.T. (1975) 'Historical notes. The past generation.' *In:* Samilson, R.L. (Ed.) *Orthopaedic Aspects of Cerebral Palsy. Clinics in Developmental Medicine No. 52/53.* London: Spastics International Medical Publications, pp. 1–4.

Johnson, D.C., Damiano, D.L., Abel, M.F. (1997) 'The evolution of gait in childhood and adolescent cerebral palsy.' *Journal of Pediatric Orthopedics*, **17**, 392–396.

Letts, M., Shapiro, L., Mulder, K., Klassen, O. (1984) 'The windblown hip syndrome in total body cerebral palsy.' *Journal of Pediatric Orthopedics*, **4**, 55–62.

Little, W.J. (1862) 'On the influence of abnormal parturition, difficult labours, premature birth and asphyxia neonatorum, on the mental and physical condition of the child, especially in relation to deformities.' *Transactions of the Obstetrical Society of London*, **3**, 293.

Miller, F., Dabney, K.W., Rang, M. (1995) 'Complications in cerebral palsy treatment.' *In:* Epps, C.H., Bowen, J.R. (Eds.) *Complications in Pediatric Orthopaedic Surgery.* Philadelphia: J.B. Lippincott, pp. 477–544.

Rang, M. (1966) *Anthology of Orthopaedics.* Edinburgh: Livingstone.

Rang, M. (1990) 'Cerebral palsy.' *In:* Morrissy, R.T. (Ed.) *Lovell and Winter's Pediatric Orthopedics, 3rd Edn.* Philadelphia: J.B. Lippincott, pp. 465–506.

Rodda, J., Graham, H.K. (2001) 'Classification of gait patterns in spastic hemiplegia and spastic diplegia: a basis for a management algorithm.' *European Journal of Neurology*, **8** (Suppl. 5), 98–108.

Salter, R.B., Field, P. (1960) 'The effects of continuous compression on living articular cartilage. An experimental investigation.' *Journal of Bone and Joint Surgery, American Volume*, **42**, 31–49.

Scrutton, D., Baird, G. (1997) 'Surveillance measures of the hips of children with bilateral cerebral palsy.' *Archives of Disease in Childhood*, **76**, 381–384.

Scrutton, D., Baird, G., Smeeton, N. (2001) 'Hip dysplasia in bilateral cerebral palsy: incidence and natural history in children aged 18 months to 5 years.' *Developmental Medicine and Child Neurology*, **43**, 586–600.

Silver, R.L., de la Garza, J., Rang, M. (1985) 'The myth of muscle balance. A study of relative strengths and excursions of normal muscles about the foot and ankle.' *Journal of Bone and Joint Surgery, British Volume*, **67**, 432–437.

Stanley, F., Blair, E., Alberman, E. (2000) *Cerebral Palsies: Epidemiology and Causal Pathways. Clinics in Developmental Medicine No 151*. London: Mac Keith Press.

Tabary, J.C., Tabary, C., Tardieu, C., Tardieu, G., Goldspink, G. (1972) 'Physiological and structural changes in the cat's soleus muscle due to immobilization at different lengths by plaster casts.' *Journal of Physiology*, **224**, 231–244.

Wiley, M.E., Damiano, D.L. (1998) 'Lower-extremity strength profiles in spastic cerebral palsy.' *Developmental Medicine and Child Neurology*, **40**, 100–107.

Williams, P.E., Goldspink, G. (1978) 'Changes in sarcomere length and physiological properties in immobilized muscle.' *Journal of Anatomy*, **127**, 459–468.

Winters, T.F., Gage, J.R., Hicks, R. (1987) 'Gait patterns in spastic hemiplegia in children and young adults.' *Journal of Bone and Joint Surgery, American Volume*, **69**, 437–441.

Ziv, I., Blackburn, N., Rang, M., Koreska, J. (1984) 'Muscle growth in normal and spastic mice.' *Developmental Medicine and Child Neurology*, **26**, 94–99.

9
THE MANAGEMENT OF DEFORMITY

Sheila McNeill

For most children with cerebral palsy (CP) there is always the prospect of musculoskeletal deformity which can have severe effects on children already severely compromised by neurological disability. It presents a major challenge to the physical management team.

The previous chapter has already described the mechanisms causing deformity and some of the surgical responses; this chapter describes the impact of deformity on the child and the rationale behind conservative intervention to prevent, minimize or reduce it. Where function is achievable, prevention of deformity may not be a priority. Thus the occurrence of some deformity should not be seen as treatment failure since it may have been significantly reduced by treatment or other treatment aims may rightly have taken priority. Where deformity has occurred, orthopaedic surgery may be needed, accompanied by physical management if the optimal benefits are to be achieved and maintained.

The problems caused by deformities

Limited range of motion at any joint restricts movement opportunities, and in CP, where movement choices are already suboptimal, it can exacerbate the disability profoundly and lead to a number of secondary problems.

SECONDARY DEFORMITY

By altering posture and movement, deformity at one joint may cause deformity at another. For instance, by effectively increasing leg length, equinus can induce compensatory hip and knee flexion. Equinus on its own is not usually difficult to correct, but the secondary fixed flexion of the hip and knee will make correction more complex. Kyphosis, associated with sacral sitting, means that the child's head will be looking downwards and so requires hyperextension of the cervical spine to compensate. This is not only difficult and uncomfortable but also leads to a shortening of the extensor soft tissue and fixed cervical lordosis.

POSTURAL STABILITY

Maintaining static or dynamic balance is compromised as postural adjustments are restricted and can be further disrupted by any misalignment of the body that shifts the line of gravity from the centre of the base. This can severely compromise sitting, standing and locomotion. In particular, asymmetric disorders cause structural asymmetry, and in quadriplegia asymmetry of the spine and hips ('windswept hips') creates an unstable trunk having only an asymmetrical and reduced base of support to balance upon. The incidence of scoliosis in ambulatory children with CP is 7% and in non-ambulatory children 39%, with the highest incidence in individuals with spastic quadriplegia (Samilson 1981).

PAIN

The prevention and treatment of pain or discomfort is a priority, and deformity is a frequent cause. Pain comes about in several ways: by restricting the postural choice a child may sit bearing too much pressure on certain areas for example on one ischial tuberosity from an asymmetric pelvis, or against the backrest upon the mid-dorsal spine from a kyphosis.

It is estimated that about one-third to one-half of children with dislocated hips have pain (Fixsen 1994). Severity of pain may be related to the degree of subluxation. The incidence of hip abnormality in individuals with CP is higher in more severely involved children (Cornell 1995), and one-third of children with a bilateral disorder have a subluxing hip by age 5 years (Scrutton *et al.* 2001). Fixsen also noted that children who continue to ambulate with a subluxed or dislocated hip are at risk of developing degenerative joint disease later in life.

FUNCTION

By preventing a full repertoire of movements, deformity will limit function. A child's hand may be almost entirely prevented from use by a fully flexed wrist; consistent eye contact is impossible with a kyphotic spine; and upper-limb use requires a well-positioned and stable trunk and base of support from the lower limbs.

GAIT

During normal gait, energy efficiency is kept to a maximum optimized by the integration of balance, muscle power generation and absorption, and sufficient range of joint movement. In ambulatory children with CP, changes in biomechanical alignment, weakness and the presence of pain result in decreased walking ability (Aronson *et al.* 1991, Johnson *et al.* 1997). Walking is an efficient means of locomotion, but it can rapidly become inefficient if deformity restricts the movement of any lower-limb joint or distorts the trunk. For example, equinus in stance phase will prevent the use of the ankle movements required for dynamic balance, forward translation of the body over the base and the power generation in the calf required for 'push-off'. Heel strike is impossible and step length is reduced. Bilateral fixed flexion at the knee causes a crouched posture throughout the gait cycle, which is not just inefficient, but requires incessant and powerful contraction of the quadriceps to remain erect.

CARE

Deformity makes the management of children with severe CP more difficult. Fixed hip adduction prevents adequate perineal hygiene, and dressing, bathing, seating and transfers are all compromised (Pope *et al.* 1991).

COSMESIS

How one looks is important and never more so than for teenagers. Visible deformity of any type affects one's view of oneself and that of the peer group. It is hard enough not moving like your friends without thinking that, in their eyes, you might also look different.

The severity of deformity

The significance of deformity varies widely from being so severe that it dominates daily life and is the major factor in treatment, to being a minor adjunct to the disability, hardly affecting the child's function now or in the likely foreseeable future.

The term 'deformity' is used to describe two quite different situations:
(1) preferred postures, often described as 'dynamic' (because they occur with attempted movement) or 'postural' (because they are always present); these deformities are not 'fixed', that is, there is still a full range of movement
(2) what are usually called 'contractures', where there is a shortening of muscle, tendon and frequently all other soft tissue, preventing a full range of movement at a joint.

Very often the two types coexist. The borderline between fixed and dynamic contractures is not always clear, with a greater range of movement often being achieved under anaesthetic. From a treatment point of view the difference is great as a postural deformity may be corrected by applying a force to the body. Thus an equinus deformity that is postural may be corrected by an ankle–foot orthosis (AFO) allowing heel strike and a good approximation to normal knee and hip posture. Obviously this is not possible with soft-tissue contracture.

Mild deformity can be one that is primarily dynamic wherein there is no or only minimal contracture. However, if the child uses this abnormal stereotyped position persistently, contracture can develop.

Moderate deformity affects passive and active motion to a larger extent and is more likely to be combined with contracture. Movement away from the direction of the deformity will be difficult and may be made harder by an increase in more generalized muscle activity. The position of the joints above and below may be compromised, causing a significant increase in the energy cost of walking (Winter 1983). Motions at adjacent joints may be coupled biomechanically due to tightness of two-joint muscles (Baddar *et al.* 2002), *e.g.* in the case of developing contracture in the gastrocnemius–soleus muscle, use of an AFO to eliminate plantarflexion may force the knee into greater crouch.

Severe deformity involves not just the muscle tendon unit, but all soft-tissue structures related to them including changes in the associated joint and bone shape. Such deformities jeopardise the child's mobility and posture, cause discomfort and sometimes pain, and often lead to severe secondary deformities. For many of these children, prevention of such deformity has to be one of the primary aims of treatment.

In my experience many children present with deformities of varying severity at multiple joints with interplay of one deformity with another. Assessment may reveal one joint or muscle group as the primary problem, and attention to this one problem may have the effect of reducing dynamic and postural deformity elsewhere. Although it is a very variable disorder, there are patterns of posture and progressions of deformity associated with various types and severities of CP that allow the prediction of problems and an opportunity for focused intervention to control the onset or progression of deformity (see Chapter 8).

Rationale for conservative treatment

The bulk of evidence for therapeutic intervention for the management of deformity in CP is empirical, although some scientific evidence exists. Many empirical methods, refined over the years, are retained because their validity and convenience are self-evident. Evidence-based research is hampered by the complexity of the problems experienced by children with CP, small or heterogenous sample sizes, and the potential ethical problems of carrying out randomized controlled trials.

Conservative treatment has been influenced by evidence on the effects of growth, muscle imbalance and effects of positioning in CP. The following are a few examples of research upon which therapy can be based.

GROWTH

The musculoskeletal status of children with CP is normal at birth (Sauser *et al.* 1986). Potential for deformity progresses with growth as spastic muscle (albeit in an animal model) grows more slowly than normal muscle in relation to bony growth (Ziv *et al.* 1984). This race between bone and muscle growth is concluded only at skeletal maturity (Boyd and Graham 1997). Intervention to counteract the progression of deformity is concentrated mostly during the period of growth. Deformity may progress after that time, however, when other factors continue to have an effect such as reduced activity and increased weight.

MUSCLE IMBALANCE
Muscle overactivity

Findings on the mechanical properties of muscle fibres from patients with spasticity have implications for conservative therapy that highlight the need for intervention to maintain normal muscle length and achieve optimum biomechanical advantage of that muscle.

According to Tardieu *et al.* (1988), stretching a hypertonic gastrocnemius–soleus muscle for more than six hours a day prevents the progression of contracture, while stretch for less than two hours a day permits its occurrence. Muscle tension is directly proportional to the amount of filament overlap (Huxley 1969); therefore an increase in the number of sarcomeres in series would be desirable in the presence of threatening contracture. Relevant to this is the ability of muscle to respond to prolonged stretch by adding more sarcomeres in series (Ziv *et al.* 1984). Denervated cat soleus muscle immobilized in the lengthened position for a period of four weeks was found to produce 25% more sarcomeres in series, while muscle immobilized in the shortened position for the same period lost 35%. This adaptation was essentially the same as in muscles that had been immobilized but not denervated (Goldspink *et al.* 1974).

More recent evidence suggests that human spastic muscle cells may be shorter and stiffer with differences in resting sarcomere length (Friden and Lieber 2003).

The disproportionate growth of tendonous components in response to stretch was demonstrated using animal studies (Wright and Rang 1990), and may provide an explanation for the condition of patella alta.

Collectively, these findings provide some guidance as to the desired cumulative effect of any treatment to impose stretch on shortened muscle.

Muscle underactivity

Muscle weakness can be a significant problem for the child with CP (Giuliani 1991, Damiano and Abel 1998). The potential for muscle weakness to lead to deformity has implications for the use of strengthening to counteract deformity. Damiano *et al.* (1995) demonstrated the effect of specific quadriceps strengthening in children with spastic diplegia. Improvement included a significant reduction of crouch gait and improvement in walking efficiency.

Shortland *et al.* (2002) suggested that fixed muscle contracture may be caused by reduced contraction of the aponeurosis due to decreased muscle-fibre diameter and that preventing such changes in muscle length through strengthening and/or electrical stimulation may be more valuable than stretching or serial casting in improving joint position.

POSITIONING

Inherently unstable structures such as the spine require good selective control to allow symmetrical development. In the absence of controlled muscle activity, external forces may override any interventions with the onset of scoliosis, as observed in paralytic conditions such as spinal muscular atrophy or acquired paraplegia. It is likely that any spasticity will further accentuate this deformity. The windswept posture in children with CP may be caused by the effect of gravity on an immobile growing child, rather than spasticity or muscle power imbalance (Scrutton and Gilbertson 1975, Fulford and Brown 1976). Therefore, asymmetrical deformity should theoretically be amenable to therapeutic positioning (Scrutton 1978). This is particularly suitable for those with a profound disability and little movement repertoire of their own.

The conservative management of deformity

THE ROLE OF THE THERAPIST

The rationale described may be translated into a treatment programme appropriate to children of various ages and levels of severity of CP. The research findings, along with a substantial empirical evidence base, indicate that management of the whole child in all situations throughout the day is appropriate in attempting to prevent disadvantageous stereotyped postures. The programme should ideally become a lifestyle (Scrutton 1984, Pope 1992).

The therapist has a major role in controlling deformity. Treatment should aim to maintain range of movement and alignment by using strategies to control the influence of deformity in various functional contexts. Specialized equipment has been developed in order to offer all-day management. None of these should be used in isolation, but rather in sequence or in conjunction with each other (De Luca 1996). The therapist needs to invest time in working with the child and her/his carers to educate them on the dangers of progressive deformity and the importance of working to avoid, where feasible, deforming activities. The therapist should assess how the child performs various functional tasks, which may show which activities reinforce the deforming postures. A child may lie down to undress quickly, allowing abnormal patterns of extension and flexion to be utilized to achieve removal of clothing. The adjustment in practice of sitting to undress may encourage the use of balance in sitting and the removal of clothing using weight transfer to either side which achieves more rotation and fewer pathological synergies. Treatment recommendations must appreciate the importance of function and self-reliance for the child.

In my experience, however, the control of deformity takes on less importance to the child when there is motivation to access opportunities involving activity. Children with moderate CP are often capable of coping independently with many functional tasks given suitable conditions and equipment. However, such children are particularly prone to the progression of deformity through the repeated use of stereotyped patterns of movement to achieve function. Such progression may then cause deterioration in functional independence as the range of movement required to perform tasks is lost. The therapist must aim for optimum intervention with flexibility to allow the child some freedom and choice. Rigid programmes are less likely to be adhered to and the therapist should show respect for the desire of an individual to pursue a variety of activities and achieve independence.

There is a need for long-term commitment from therapists, carers and the individual to protect the body from deformity (Goldsmith 2000). A significant concentration of thera-peutic effort is directed to children, but as Bottos *et al*. (2001) have pointed out, contact with health and rehabilitative services is radically reduced on reaching adulthood; these authors also recommended a more independence-orientated therapeutic approach.

Thus, the evidence we have shows that to prevent deformity the body tissues need to move through their full range and not be allowed to maintain favoured postures for long periods; while to correct or control deformity, prolonged periods away from the favoured position are needed. This can be achieved in a number of ways, and the method of choice is often governed by the degree of deformity and the functional ability of the child. The means are: (1) muscle strengthening, (2) reducing hypertonia, (3) static equipment, (4) serial casting, and (5) orthoses.

The management of children with profound CP and the likelihood of deformity present a challenge to the therapist whose ultimate goal must be to ensure that intervention to control deformity improves the child's quality of life. In some instances, this may imply being able to do little more than ensuring they are more easily cared for and comfortable.

These children require regular changes in position as they have very little or no ability to change position themselves within their external support (Bell and Watson 1985). No matter how well equipment positions a child, change in position is necessary to maintain joint range and relieve pressure. Particular attention to spinal posture should feature in the general handling of all these children, as relatively minor deteriorations in spinal posture may have an adverse general impact on the child's disability (Scrutton and Gilbertson 1975).

Children with profound CP and multiple deformities frequently experience difficulty with positioning for feeding, washing, perineal hygiene, relaxation and stimulation. Also, these children may experience pain or discomfort. They require a programme of management that involves the parents and carers working together, providing appropriate handling to contain and counteract where possible the child's deformity. At the same time the programme must include attention to the secondary problems encountered by the child such as feeding difficulties, reflux, poor vision/hearing, epilepsy, respiratory problems, digestive problems, renal problems and problems of circulation, any of which can affect the postural programme.

MUSCLE STRENGTHENING

Muscle weakness has now been recognized as a significant problem for many children with CP.

Exercises

Strengthening may be achieved in a functional context such as practising sit to stand, or in a more specific way such as quadriceps strengthening using resisted exercise (Damiano *et al.* 1995).

Electrical stimulation

Over the past 15 years there has been an increase in the number of reports documenting the effects of various types of electrical stimulation in children with CP. Electrical stimulation has been utilized in muscle strengthening (Dubowitz *et al.* 1988, Hazlewood *et al.* 1994), increasing joint range of movement (Hazlewood *et al.* 1994) and improving gross and fine motor skills (Steinbok *et al.* 1997, Wright and Granat 2000) in this patient group. As yet there is no consensus as to which treatment parameters are most effective and which patient population the most suitable for this type of intervention.

REDUCING HYPERTONIA

Theoretically the use of localized intramuscular botulinum toxin A or the systemic use of oral or intrathecal baclofen has the potential to prevent contractures by reducing hypertonia, thereby allowing greater ease of active or passive movement. The use of these therapies is discussed in Chapter 7.

STATIC EQUIPMENT

Positioning in lying

The control of prone, supine and alternate side-lying positioning is essential in the management of the child to avoid or delay the onset of spinal and hip deformity.

In supine, a T-roll under the knees is used to stabilize the pelvis better. The vertical arm of the roll separates the legs; the horizontal arm maintains knee and so hip flexion, decreasing lumbar lordosis (Pope 1992).

A side-lying board provides an alternative to the flexed sitting position, is less demanding for the child with profound CP than the use of a prone stander, and can be adapted to counteract lateral postural spinal curvature.

Sleeping posture

Orthotic systems for controlling sleeping posture have been developed to provide comfortable and versatile support for those unable to move during sleep. With adequate support, optimum symmetry is possible (Goldsmith 2000). The child lies on a pressure-relieving surface and is supported by a series of brackets and cushions that is built around the body holding the child in a corrected position (Fig. 9.1). The even weight distribution in supported lying minimizes the risk of tissue trauma (Pountney *et al.* 2000).

Hankinson and Morton (2002) demonstrated in a pilot study the use of a sleeping

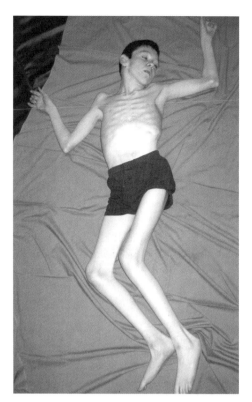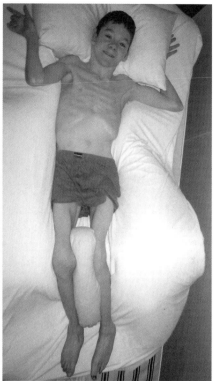

Fig. 9.1. A 14-year-old boy with severe spastic quadriplegia who assumes a windswept position in supine *(left)* is brought into a more symmetrical position with the support of a sleeping system *(right)*.

system that reduced hip subluxation by providing hip abduction during sleep.

The family requires training and support from their therapist on the use and review of the system (Goldsmith 2000).

Seating

Specialized seating may be required for children with severe CP to give complete support, comfort and control of progressing deformities (Fig. 9.2). The development of switches attached to seating and appropriate computer software has enabled many children with profound disability to access information technology to communicate, avail themselves of teaching resources and record their work.

Seating systems can address the problems of inadequate balance and postural instability and have the potential to maintain position sufficient to allow optimum function without development of deformity (Pope *et al*. 1988). Pelvic stability in anterior pelvic tilt is essential, with a stable, symmetric position that helps to prevent an undesirable increase in tonus (Pope *et al*. 1988).

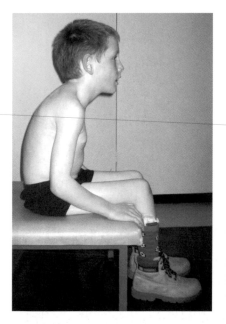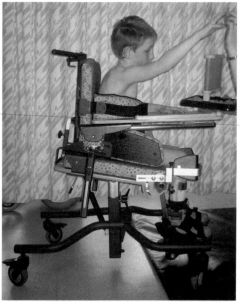

Fig. 9.2. A 9-year-old boy with severe spastic quadriplegia and insufficient trunk stability to permit upper-limb function in bench sitting *(left)*, is seated in a forward-leaning position with anterior pelvic tilt *(right)*, encouraging trunk extension and the possibility of upper-limb function.

Children with severe CP may require trunk support to control adverse spinal movements and a wide distribution of body weight to maintain tissue integrity (Pope *et al.* 1988). Seating assessment should include attention to the impact of orientation on the child's general tone. EMG studies demonstrated that both back extensors and hip adductors show a significant increase in tone in the tilted position relative to the vertical position (Nwaobi 1986). The 'high guard' position with retracted shoulders frequently assumed in the reclined position compromises the potential for upper-limb function as the child cannot bring the hands to midline (Nwaobi 1987).

Pope *et al.* (1988) described four positions that may help the child with CP to achieve postural stability in sitting:
(1) upright posture
(2) forward lean—anterior trunk support provided by arms resting on a wedge placed on a tray
(3) backward tilt—with head supported in flexion for horizontal vision
(4) straddle combined with forward lean—a straddle seat fixes the pelvis and trunk support is anterior. This seating requires some postural ability to maintain position with support.

Standing frames
The judicious use of standing frames may be of potential benefit to children with both

138

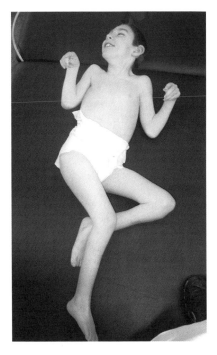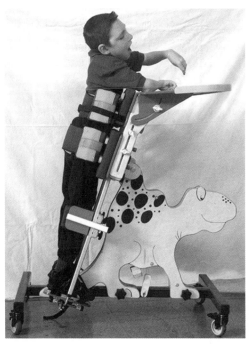

Fig. 9.3. A 10-year-old boy with severe spastic quadriplegia, who assumes a windswept position in supine *(left)*, is brought into an improved symmetrical position with the help of a prone stander *(right)*. This gives the possibility of active trunk extension and upper-limb function.

profound and moderate CP. The standing frame provides an obvious change of position for a non-ambulant child (Fig. 9.3). It provides a good application of the goal of achieving prolonged periods of stretch and in this way helps to delay or prevent the onset of deformity (Stuberg 1992).

Activity away from deforming flexed postures is desirable. An essential element of any standing position is the plantigrade positioning of the feet, forming the base upon which the child's body is supported. Where foot deformity is present, these need to be accommodated to ensure correct weight bearing through the long axes of the lower limbs.

Normally the acetabulum and the femoral head develop congruently. External loads of muscle tension and weight bearing guide this development if applied through the neutral angle of lower limbs (LeVeau and Bernhardt 1984, Stuberg 1992). If the femoral head is centralized in the hip joint early (by 4 years old) the hip joint will be less likely to sublux or dislocate (Kalen and Bleck 1985, Scrutton and Baird 1997).

Upright standers are also used in the management of smaller children to allow access to play activities (Fig. 9.4).

The development of motorized sit-to-stand equipment has provided a safe means to achieve an upright position. These are becoming essential to protect carers in the management of many children with disabilities.

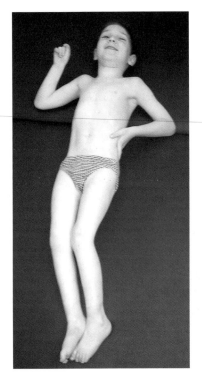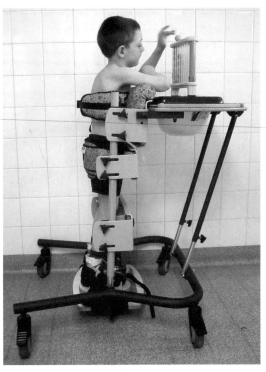

Fig. 9.4. An 8-year-old boy with severe spastic quadriplegia, who assumes a windswept position in supine *(left)*, is brought into a more upright position in an upright stander *(right)*. Trunk support may be reduced, and this has the potential benefit of positioning at a regular table in the classroom.

SERIAL CASTING

Upper limbs

Some work has been carried out to demonstrate the effect of serial casting on upper limbs, including elbow and wrist flexion, and forearm pronation deformities (Yasukawa and Sisung 1990, Steer 1989). Steer reported on six single case studies. All the children demonstrated an increased range of movement, and although none achieved maximum range of movement, all showed an increased freedom of movement. The range of movement gained was usually reversed by six months, indicating a need for regular re-casting. Steer advocated a post-casting regime of upper-limb night splints and twice daily applications of bivalved casts for two hours during the day.

Lower limbs

Serial casting has been widely used in the treatment of dynamic or mild fixed equinus deformity in children with CP, which causes the characteristic inefficient toe-walking gait (Tardieu *et al*. 1982, Brouwer *et al*. 1998, Cottalorda *et al*. 2000). It has also been applied to the knee to treat hamstrings/knee flexion contracture (Phillips and Audet 1990).

The aim of this treatment on an equinus deformity is to gain a plantigrade foot, prevent skeletal deformity and improve gait (Cottalorda *et al*. 2000).

Such casting is beneficial to the young child with CP as a way of delaying the need for surgery. Surgical intervention at this stage is not advised due to the delayed maturation of the CNS characteristic of CP, which may produce unpredictable and variable results (Graham and Fixsen 1988). If surgery is indicated at a later stage, lengthening can then be undertaken on an unscarred tendon (Cottalorda *et al*. 2000). Failure to regain range of movement using serial casting is one indicator to proceed to surgical lengthening (DeLuca 1996).

Protocols for this treatment vary slightly. An example is that of Cottalorda *et al*. (2000), who applied casts weekly over a total of three weeks to treat equinus successfully. Casting is not an isolated therapy, but as part of the whole package of measures including physical therapy and orthotics used to manage equinus deformity in small children (Cottalorda *et al*. 2000).

Several researchers have studied the effects of botulinum toxin A (BTX-A) in conjunction with or as an alternative to serial casting. Flett *et al*. (1999) found that BTX-A injections were of similar efficacy to serial casts in improving dynamic equinus in ambulant or partially ambulant children. Desloovere *et al*. (2001) studied the combined effect of BTX-A and serial casting, and found more prolonged improvements in children who were cast immediately after multilevel BTX-A injections, as opposed to those who were cast before injections. The use of BTX-A is further discussed in Chapter 7.

ORTHOTICS

Orthoses are useful in the management of deformity because they apply a sustained stretch to a hypertonic muscle/tendon group and by positioning one joint can gain better posture and muscle activity elsewhere. Orthoses may be articulated to allow movement about a specific joint, thereby allowing muscles to be more active (Burtner *et al*. 1999).

Upper limbs

Information about the effects of the many designs of upper-limb orthoses is limited and equivocal. There is little doubt that in theory orthoses should be effective but there are practical problems. The hand movements are too fine and the lever arms so short that anything but rather crude hand splints are difficult to use; and control of the wrist and elbow can limit function too greatly. It is easier to treat the most profoundly disabled children because, lacking fine movement, controlling the posture of the wrist and fingers is not difficult. For these children, preventing wrist and finger flexion deformities is of great importance to make their care easier and prevent low-grade palmar infection.

Trunk

The treatment of scoliosis by plastic body jackets may provide an adjunct to stability or act as an extended lever arm for the pelvis to control the hips.

Hips

Bower (1990) addressed the problem of potential hip deformity by developing, with a team

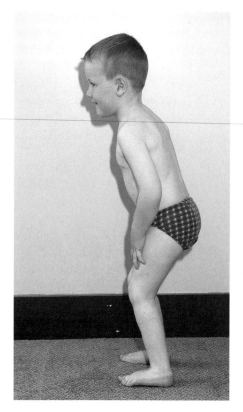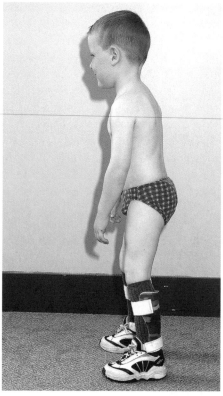

Fig. 9.5. A 3-year-old boy with spastic diplegia who experiences crouched posture in standing *(left)*, is brought into a more upright position with the application of rigid ankle–foot orthoses *(right)*.

of orthotists, a hip abduction and spinal orthosis made out of polypropylene components with rigid metal side bars and flexion/extension hinges at the hips to allow the child to sit, stand and lie in the orthosis. The spinal jacket holds the spine perpendicular to the horizontally aligned hips. Thigh cuffs hold the hips in about 30° of abduction, with an adjustable abduction bar positioned between the thigh cuffs. Although the author has no experience of this orthosis, the approach of such corrected positioning seems logical if tolerated by the child.

Lower limbs
Potential deformity may be prevented or reduced with the appropriate use of orthoses. Static orthoses for night have been broadly accepted as useful for maintaining corrected joint positions during sleep. These include the knee orthosis, ankle–foot orthosis and knee–ankle–foot orthosis. Lower-limb daytime orthoses for the ambulant child prevent deformity by aiming to bring the child's gait to within normal parameters, providing improved alignment and movement through more normal ranges (Figs. 9.5, 9.6).

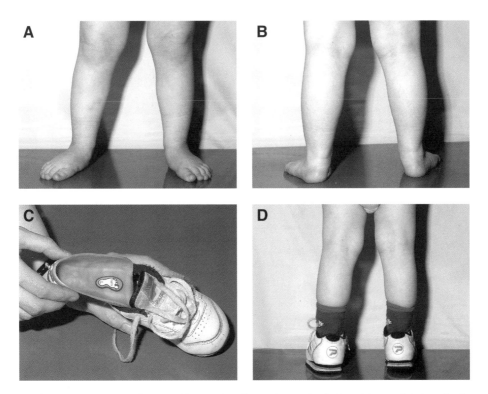

Fig. 9.6. A 3-year-old boy with general hypotonia and emerging ataxia who is unable to walk independently (A,B), with use of UCBL(University of California at Berkeley Laboratory) insoles inserted into his shoes to stabilize the subtalar joints (C), has gained sufficient stability to walk independently (D).

Recommendations for gait orthotics are made based on the biomechanical ability of a given device to improve gait as described in terms of five principles outlined by Gage (1991): (1) stability during stance; (2) sufficient foot clearance during swing; (3) prepositioning of the foot at the end of swing; (4) adequate stride length; (5) energy efficiency.

When assessing how appropriate an orthosis is for a child, the team must consider it in terms of each of these principles in order to optimize the effect of any prescription.

Conclusion

An appreciation of the consequences of deformity and the potential of prevention and correction has a strong influence on management strategies for children with CP. This involves a coordinated package of ongoing care requiring liaison between the child/ parents/carers/teachers and the child's therapists, paediatrician, orthopaedic surgeon and orthotist. Where communication is effective, advice is consistent and input is more likely to be received with confidence and introduced into the child's routine.

Children grow and circumstances change, so for an optimum effect, regular assessment of the current treatment is needed. There is also a responsibility to use and produce 'scientific' evidence on which to base an evolving practice for the general population of children with CP.

ACKNOWLEDGEMENTS

I would like to thank the therapy staff in Fleming Fulton and Mitchell House Schools, Belfast, and staff in the Gait Analysis Laboratory, Musgrave Park Hospital, Belfast, for their help in compiling this chapter.

REFERENCES

Aronson, D.D., Zak, P.J., Lee, C.L., Bollinger, R.O., Lamont, R.L. (1991) 'Posterior transfer of the adductors in children who have cerebral palsy.' *Journal of Bone and Joint Surgery, American Volume*, **73**, 59–65.

Baddar, A., Granata, K., Damiano, D.L., Carmines, D.V., Blanco, J.S., Abel, M.F. (2002) 'Ankle and knee coupling in patients with spastic diplegia: effects of gastrocnemius–soleus lengthening.' *Journal of Bone and Joint Surgery, American Volume*, **84**, 736–744.

Bell, E., Watson, A. (1985) 'The prevention of positional deformity in cerebral palsy.' *Physiotherapy Practice*, **1**, 86–92.

Bottos, M., Feliciangeli, A., Sciuto, L., Gericke, C., Vianello, A. (2001) 'Functional status of adults with cerebral palsy and implications for treatment of children.' *Developmental Medicine and Child Neurology*, **43**, 516–528.

Boyd, R.N., Graham, H.K. (1997) 'Botulinum toxin A in the management of children with cerebral palsy: indications and outcome.' *European Journal of Neurology*, **4** (Suppl. 2), 515–522.

Bower, E. (1990) 'Hip abduction and spinal orthosis in cerebral palsy.' *Physiotherapy*, **76**, 658–659.

Brouwer, B., Wheeldon, R.K., Stradiotti-Parker, N., Allum, J. (1998) 'Reflex excitability and isometric force production in cerebral palsy: the effect of serial casting.' *Developmental Medicine and Child Neurology*, **40**, 168–175.

Burtner, P.A., Woollacott , MH.,. Qualls, C. (1999) 'Stance balance control with orthoses in a group of children with spastic cerebral palsy.' *Developmental Medicine and Child Neurology*, **41**, 748–757.

Cornell, M.S. (1995) 'The hip in cerebral palsy.' *Developmental Medicine and Child Neurology*, **37**, 3–18.

Cottalorda, J., Gautheron, V., Metton, G., Charmet, Y., Chavrier, Y. (2000) 'Toe-walking in children younger than six years with cerebral palsy.' *Journal of Bone and Joint Surgery, British Volume*, **82**, 541–544.

Damiano, D.L., Abel, M.F. (1998) 'Functional outcomes of strength training in spastic cerebral palsy.' *Archives of Physical Medicine and Rehabilitation*, **79**, 119–125.

Damiano, D.L., Kelly, L.E., Vaughan, C.L.. (1995) 'Effects of quadriceps femoris muscle strengthening on crouch gait in children with spastic diplegia.' *Physical Therapy*, **75**, 658–667.

DeLuca, P.A. (1996) 'The musculoskeletal management of children with cerebral palsy.' *Paediatric Clinics of North America*, **43**, 1135–1150.

Desloovere, K., Molenaers, G., Jonkers, I., De Cat, J., De Borre, L., Nijs, J., Eyssen, M., Pauwels, P., De Cock, P. (2001) 'A randomised study of combined botulinum toxin type A and casting in an ambulant child with cerebral palsy using objective outcome measures.' *European Journal of Neurology*, **8**, Suppl. 5, 75–87.

Dubowitz, L., Finnie, N., Hyd, S.A., Scott, O.M., Vrbova, G. (1988) 'Improvement of muscle performance by chronic electrical stimulation in children with cerebral palsy.' *Lancet*, **1**, 587–588.

Fixsen, J.A. (1994) 'Orthopaedic management of cerebral palsy.' *Archives of Disease in Childhood*, **71**, 396–397.

Flett, P.J., Stern, L.M., Waddy, H., Connell, T.M., Seeger, J.D., Gibson, S.K. (1999) 'Botulinum toxin A versus fixed cast stretching for dynamic calf tightness in cerebral palsy.' *Journal of Paediatric Child Health*, **35**, 71–77.

Friden, J., Lieber, R.L. (2003) 'Spastic muscle cells are shorter and stiffer than normal cells.' *Muscle and Nerve*, **27**, 157–164.

Fulford, G.E., Brown, J.K. (1976) 'Position as a cause of deformity in children with cerebral palsy.' *Developmental Medicine and Child Neurology*, **18**, 305–314.

Gage, J.R. (1991) *Gait Analysis in Cerebral Palsy. Clinics in Developmental Medicine No. 121.* London: Mac Keith Press.

Giuliani, C.A. (1991) 'Dorsal rhizotomy for children with cerebral palsy: support for concepts in motor control.' *Physical Therapy*, **71**, 248–259.

Goldsmith, S. (2000) 'Postural care at night within a community setting.' *Physiotherapy*, **86**, 528–534.

Goldspink, G., Tabary, C., Tabary, J.C., Tardieu, C., Tardieu, G. (1974) 'The effect of denervation on the adaptation of sarcomere number and muscle extensibility to the functional length of the muscle.' *Journal of Physiology*, 236, 733–742.

Graham, H.K., Fixsen, J.A. (1988) 'Lengthening of the calcaneal tendon in spastic hemiplegia by the white slide technique.' *Journal of Bone and Joint Surgery, British Volume*, **70**, 472–475.

Hankinson, J., Morton, R.E. (2002) 'Use of a lying hip abduction system in children with bilateral cerebral palsy: a pilot study.' *Developmental Medicine and Child Neurology*, **44**, 177–180.

Hazlewood, M.E., Brown, J.K., Rowe, P.J., Salter, P.M. (1994) 'The use of therapeutic electrical stimulation in the treatment of hemiplegic cerebral palsy.' *Developmental Medicine and Child Neurology*, 36, 661–673.

Huxley, H.E. (1969) 'The mechanism of muscular contraction.' *Science*, **164**, 1356–1366. [Reprinted in *Clinical Orthopaedics*, 2002, **403** (Suppl.), S6–S17.]

Johnson, D.C., Damiano, D.L., Abel, M.F. (1997) 'The evolution of gait in childhood and adolescent cerebral palsy.' *Journal of Pediatric Orthopedics*, **17**, 392–396.

Kalen, V., Bleck, E.E. (1985) 'Prevention of spastic paralytic dislocation of the hip.' *Developmental Medicine and Child Neurology*, **27**, 17–24.

LeVeau, B.F., Bernhardt, D.B. (1984) 'Developmental biomechanics—effect of forces on the growth, development and maintenance of the human body.' *Physical Therapy*, **64**, 1874–1882.

Nwaobi, O.M. (1986) 'Effects of body orientation in space on tonic muscle activity of patients with cerebral palsy.' *Developmental Medicine and Child Neurology*, **28**, 41–44.

Nwaobi, O.M. (1987) 'Seating orientations and upper extremity function in children with cerebral palsy.' *Physical Therapy*, **67**, 1209–1212.

Phillips, W.E., Audet, M. (1990) 'Use of serial casting in the management of knee joint contractures in an adolescent with cerebral palsy.' *Physical Therapy*, **70**, 521–523.

Pope, P.M. (1992) 'Management of the physical condition in patients with chronic and severe neurological pathologies.' *Physiotherapy*, **78**, 896–903.

Pope, P.M., Booth, E., Gosling, G. (1988) 'The development of alternative seating and mobility systems.' *Physiotherapy Practice*, **4**, 78–93.

Pope, P.M., Bowes, C.E., Tudor, M. (1991) 'Surgery combined with continuing post-operative stretching and management for knee flexion contractures in cases of multiple sclerosis – a report of six cases.' *Clinical Rehabilitation*, **5**, 15–23.

Pountney, T.E., Mulcahy, C.M., Clarke, S.M., Green, E.M. (2000) *The Chailey Approach to Postural Mangement.* Birmingham: Active Design.

Samilson, R.L. (1981) 'Orthopaedic surgery of the hips and spine in retarded cerebral palsied patients.' *Orthopaedic Clinics of North America*, **12**, 83–90.

Sauser, D.D., Hewes, R.C., Root, L. (1986) 'Hip changes in spastic cerebral palsy.' *American Journal of Roentgenology*, **146**, 1219–1222.

Scrutton, D. (1978) 'Developmental deformity and the profoundly retarded child.' *In:* Apley, J. (Ed.) *Care of the Handicapped Child. Clinics in Developmental Medicine No. 67.* London: Spastics International Medical Publications, pp. 83–84.

Scrutton, D. (1984) 'Aim oriented management.' *In:* Scrutton, D. (Ed.) *Management of the Motor Disorders of Children with Cerebral Palsy. Clinics in Developmental Medicine No. 90.* London: Spastics International Medical Publications, pp. 49–58.

Scrutton, D., Baird, G. (1997) 'Surveillance measures of the hips of children with bilateral cerebral palsy.' *Archives of Disease in Childhood*, **76**, 381–384.

Scrutton, D., Gilbertson, M. (1975) 'Movement disorders and orthopaedic situations.' *In:* Apley J. (Ed.) *Physiotherapy in Paediatric Practice.* London: Butterworths, pp. 32–58.

Scrutton, D., Baird, G., Smeeton, N. (2001) 'Hip dysplasia in bilateral cerebral palsy: incidence and natural history in children aged 18 months to 5 years.' *Developmental Medicine and Child Neurology*, **43**, 586–600.

Shortland, A.P., Harris, C.A., Gough, M., Robinson, R.O. (2002) 'Architecture of the medial gastrocnemius in children with spastic diplegia.' *Developmental Medicine and Child Neurology*, **44**, 158–164.

Steer, V. (1989) 'Upper limb serial casting i with cerebral palsy – a preliminary report.' *Australian Occupational Therapy Journal*, **36**, 69–77.

Steinbok, P., Reiner, A., Kestle, J.R.W. (1997) 'Therapeutic electrical stimulation following selective posterior rhizotomy in children with spastic diplegic cerebral palsy: a randomised controlled trial.' *Developmental Medicine and Child Neurology*, **39**, 515–520.

Stuberg, W.A. (1992) 'Considerations related to weight-bearing programs in children with developmental disabilities.' *Physical Therapy*, **72**, 35–40.

Tardieu, G., Tardieu, C., Colbeau-Justin, P., Lespargot, A. (1982) 'Muscle hypoextensibility in children with cerebral palsy. II. Therapeutic implications.' *Archives of Physical Medicine and Rehabilitation*, **63**, 103–107.

Tardieu, C., Lespargot ,A,. Tabary, C., Bret, M.D. (1988) 'For how long must the soleus muscle be stretched each day to prevent contracture?' *Developmental Medicine and Child Neurology*, **30**, 3–10.

Winter, D.A. (1983) 'Knee flexion during stance as a determinant of inefficient walking.' *Physical Therapy*, **63**, 331–333.

Wright, J., Rang, M. (1990) 'The spastic mouse: and the search for an animal model of spasticity in human beings.' *Clinical Orthopaedics and Related Research*, **253**, 12–19.

Wright, P.A., Granat, M.H. (2000) 'Therapeutic effects of functional electrical stimulation of the upper limb of eight children with cerebral palsy.' *Developmental Medicine and Child Neurology*, **42**, 724–727.

Yasukawa, A., Sisung, C. (1990) 'Upper-extremity casting: adjunct to therapy for hemiplegia secondary to cerebral palsy.' *Developmental Medicine and Child Neurology*, **32**, Suppl. 62, 3–4. *(Abstract.)*

Ziv, I., Blackburn, N., Rang, M., Koreska, J. (1984) 'Muscle growth in normal and spastic mice.' *Developmental Medicine and Child Neurology*, **26**, 94–99.

10
PHYSIOTHERAPY MANAGEMENT IN CEREBRAL PALSY: AN UPDATE ON TREATMENT APPROACHES

Margaret Mayston

Given the diversity of the effects of cerebral palsy (CP) on any individual, it is not surprising that evidence to support the positive effects of intervention is lacking (Hur 1995). Randomized controlled trials can be difficult to carry out both because of small sample sizes and for ethical reasons (Hur 1995, Reddihough *et al*. 1998), and most studies concentrate on the effects of early intervention for the high-risk groups (Weindling 2000). Overall, results are inconclusive. Despite this, therapy is widely advocated and desired and there are many approaches to the management of CP (Table 10.1). The most common named approaches are Bobath (also known as Neurodevelopmental Therapy), and Conductive Education (Peto), although most therapists would consider that they use an eclectic approach. Other approaches include Vojta (in Europe), Doman–Delacato (Institute for the Achievement of Human Potential, IAHP; British Institute for Brain Injured Children, BIBIC; Brainwave), Sensory Integration, and Movement Opportunities Via Education (MOVE), the choice and availability of which varies from country to country. The emergence of various adjuncts such as electrical stimulation, recreationally based therapies [*e.g.* hydrotherapy (aquatherapy), hippotherapy] and alternative therapies (Hurvitz *et al*. 2003) (*e.g.* acupressure, osteocranio-sacral therapy) further broadens the options available, increasing the dilemma for both families and those in the management team. Many myths surround the various therapy approaches, and new ideas seem to be constantly emerging (Logan 2002). A recent newcomer to the management options is Advance Neuromotor Rehabilitation (ANR). This approach has its origins in Russia and claims to offer a cure for CP. This is misleading and liable to be the cause of great distress to parents/families of children with CP as it is quite clear that there is no cure for CP. It may well be that in the early months following birth, especially an extremely preterm birth, some adverse signs that suggest the possibility of CP might be present, *e.g.* periods of atypical movement patterns or persistent asymmetry. However, it is generally accepted that such signs can dissipate, so that after a period of monitoring progress, the child is discharged and treatment has not been required (Nelson and Ellenberg 1982, Graves 1995).

Although there have been some attempts to evaluate effectiveness of CP management (Palmer *et al*. 1988; Bairstow *et al*. 1993; Bower *et al*. 1994, 1996, 2001; Knox and Evans 2002), little or no evidence is available to show that therapy offered by the 'named approaches' is effective or that one approach is more beneficial than another. And yet, therapy programmes

TABLE 10.1
Common therapeutic approaches to the management of CP

Bobath/Neurodevelopmental Therapy (NDT)
Conductive Education (Peto)
Sensory Integration (SI)
Patterning (Doman–Delacato, *i.e.* IAHP/BIBIC/Brainwave)
Movement Opportunities Via Education (MOVE)
Vojta
Advance Neuromotor Rehabilitation (ANR)
Hyperbaric oxygen (HBO)
Recreactional therapies, *e.g.* hippotherapy, hydrotherapy
Alternative therapies, *e.g.* acupuncture, osteocraniosacral therapy

are considered an integral part of the management of the child with CP (Flett 2003). Other questions often asked are "how much?" and "how soon?"; again for these questions there are no definitive answers (Bower *et al.* 1996, Reddihough *et al.* 1998, Weindling 2000, Bower and McLellan 2001). And yet, on the basis of what is known about central nervous system (CNS) changes during development, it would appear that early therapy should be effective in minimizing the negative effects of CP at least in some children. In addition, increasing knowledge of the underlying mechanisms of CP and possibilities for early detection should enable more effective management of the condition (Prechtl *et al.* 1997, Cioni 2002). The concept of neuroplasticity is also an attractive factor for promoting the intervention process. Given that experience seems to be important in shaping function of the developing nervous system (Hadders-Algra *et al.* 1996, Hadders-Algra 2001), therapy should have a significant effect on quality of outcome. The availability of measurement tools gives the possibility of determining what might be the most effective intervention (see Chapters 4 and 5).

The main aim of therapy for the child with CP should be to improve the quality of life for the individual person and their family, to maximize their potential for participation in daily life activities, and to prepare for improved quality of life during adult years. Depending on the age of the child and severity of the disability three general aims can be identified (Mayston 2001): (1) maintain functional level, (2) increase or improve the skill repertoire, (3) general management and minimisation of contractures and deformities.

It is beyond the scope of this chapter to cover all approaches, but the most commonly encountered ones will be reviewed, recognizing of course that each is rarely applied in its 'pure' form. It is also recognized that research shows that no one particular approach is better than another, nor is the basis of any one approach clearly understood. The fact that the originators of Bobath, Conductive Education and Sensory Integration are no longer alive further complicates matters as their approaches have been changed and modified in different ways in different places.

Common approaches

BOBATH

The Bobaths summarized their approach (which they introduced in the 1940s) concisely in the first edition of this book (Bobath and Bobath 1984). The Bobath approach is known in some countries (*e.g.* USA, South Africa and some European countries) as Neurodevelopmental Therapy. There are thousands of Bobath-trained therapists and teachers of Bobath throughout the world, but great diversity exists among them according to when they trained, with whom they trained and to what extent they incorporate other modalities, *e.g.* electrical stimulation and strength training. This means that a therapist in one country who is called 'Bobath trained' may practise in a quite different way from their counterpart in another country or who trained many years earlier or with a different tutor. The understanding of the approach is further confounded by the lack of publications, and the lack of detail in existing publications on the specific type of programme implemented. Now that the original proponents are no longer alive, many people have 'developed' the approach and it is not clear at times exactly what Bobath has become.

The Bobaths emphasized that it was an approach or concept not a method, and is primarily a way of thinking. Therapists are trained to be multi/transdisciplinary, *i.e.* physiotherapists, occupational therapists, speech therapists and language therapists train together and work towards achieving common goals, sharing core skills of assessment and management. The approach recognizes that all people with neurodisability have potential for enhanced function (*i.e.* neuroplasticity of the CNS). To optimize function and participation, there is recognition of an ongoing need for a thorough analysis of the child's functional skills from motor, sensory, perceptual, cognitive and musculoskeletal perspectives. It claims to emphasize a realistic approach; Bobath stressed that the goal should be to work for what the person could do with a little help, *i.e.* that which was necessary for the person and difficult but not impossible to achieve. Although the therapy has been viewed as being too passive (Carr and Shepherd 1998), Bobath emphasized the need for the person's own more effective activity and repetition for learning. To achieve this, therapists train parents and carers in ways to assist their child to achieve best performance, learning to remove the assistance when possible. One of the emphases has been on the life-long nature of the condition of CP, and, as such, the Bobath therapist is forward looking to the quality of adult life, emphasizing the need to minimize deformity, recognizing the need for good positioning in equipment, the use of orthotics, and the use of adjuncts such as botulinum toxin and surgery as appropriate. This is more critical in the current population of children with CP who are observed to have an element of hypotonia and weakness underlying their spastic hypertonia (Mayston 2001). Current UK courses teach an approach that as much as possible is based on available knowledge and evidence and recognizes the outmoded nature of aiming to inhibit abnormal reflexes and placing the emphasis on facilitating postural reactions; however, this is not necessarily so in other countries.

The Bobath approach suggests that normal or near-normal muscle tone (currently both neural and non-neural aspects are considered: Mayston 2002) is essential as a basis for effective movement to carry out activities of daily life. Therapists use ways of handling, positioning and guiding movement that improve quality of tone and movement; these techniques are taught to parents and carers and incorporated into activities of daily life to optimize participation. These techniques are used in conjunction with positioning, orthotics, use of equipment (*e.g.* standing frames, specialized seating), judicious use of surgery, agents such as botulinum toxin, and other modalities, *e.g.* lycra orthoses. Parents, child and therapists

149

determine goals in partnership to maximize functional potential and to improve the quality of life for adulthood. Although the emphasis is on motor abilities, the approach also recognizes that other factors such as sensory, perceptual and cognitive function might be the major factors limiting participation in everyday activities.

The Bobaths suggested that not all activities of development are essential (*e.g.* many children walk without ever crawling), but stressed the key components that form the basis for skilled activity against gravity. The term 'preparation for function' is used (stretching tight muscles, practise of task components), but this preparation must be translated into the activity prepared for, *e.g.* extension of hips for standing, and then practise of standing. Well coordinated teamwork is considered to be essential, and therapists are trained to be transdisciplinary as well as multidisciplinary and to manage the individual in an holistic manner. For example, the physiotherapist may sometimes work on hand function, often considered the domain of the occupational therapist, but will also call on the special expertise of the appropriate discipline when necessary. Individual programmes are devised and taught to all people in the child's life where possible, although the principles of the Bobath approach can be applied in a group setting. All children are treated regardless of age and severity.

Therapy provision at the UK Bobath centres is intensive (daily sessions for two weeks), consultative, and in a few cases is provided on a regular basis. Outcome measures are being used to determine the effects of therapy at those centres (Knox and Evans 2002), and have also been used to determine the efficacy of the approach or aspects of it, but there is no conclusive evidence to show that it is effective or what elements of the Bobath/NDT approach are most beneficial (Palmer *et al.* 1988; for a review, see Butler and Darrah 2001).

As an approach, like all of the other named and established approaches, Bobath does not provide a total management package for children with CP, and on its own cannot meet all children's needs. The emphasis on tone management has perhaps meant that areas such as muscle strength and biomechanics, now known to be significant impairments in CP and which can be effectively changed with the appropriate intervention (Damiano *et al.* 1998), have been neglected by Bobath therapists. However, the emphasis of handling and positioning to optimize the limited functional capacity of the child is valued by parents and carers, especially for the more severely multiply disabled child.

CONDUCTIVE EDUCATION (PETO)

Around the same time as the Bobaths started their work, Conductive Education (CE) was being developed in Budapest, Hungary, by Prof. Andreas Peto (details of the approach can be read in the first edition, Hári and Tillemans 1984). He, like the Bobaths, is no longer alive, and others have taken on the responsibility of promoting the approach and developing its use throughout the world, especially in the UK and Australia. As with Bobath/NDT, CE has been altered from its original form and changed to adapt it to be more compatible with the daily life routine. The approach was originally introduced primarily to teach children to walk, a prerequisite for attendance at school in Hungary at that time. The intervention was carried out in a residential group setting, with the whole day organized to promote independence. Although CE is viewed by many as a therapy approach, its proponents are very clear that this is not the case: it is primarily a learning process. Thus CE approaches the problems of movement as problems of learning (a philosophy shared with the Movement Opportunities Via Education).

CE is based on the idea that children with motor disabilities develop and learn in the same way as their peers, and this of course requires a certain level of cognitive ability to be successful. Children learn to function by integrating cognitive, emotional, social, sensori-motor and communication skills into a meaningful whole. It is viewed as a simple process. It emphasizes participation in whatever way the child can manage, and there is no complicated equipment to facilitate motor control and stability. The use of plinths, ladder-back chairs and simple orthotics is all that is required.

CE is usually carried out in a group educational setting with school-age children, although early intervention is provided in the form of mother/toddler groups with the idea that education must be started as early as possible. Whereas the multidisciplinary approach favoured by the traditional and Bobath systems recognizes differences in specialist knowledge about the child, the Conductor is trained to facilitate all aspects of the child's development. The emphasis is on development of independence with all children working according to the best of their abilities, irrespective of movement quality. The advantage of the approach is its emphasis on the child's initiation, participation and practise in daily activities in the most efficient way that they can. This is the major factor that distinguishes it from the Bobath approach, which emphasizes the quality of function and its relevance to future development.

A comparative study of traditional therapy versus CE showed little difference between outcomes, but more contractures were present in the CE group (Bairstow *et al.* 1993, Reddihough *et al.* 1998).

SENSORY INTEGRATION
Sensory integration (SI) is a conceptual model of therapy practice originally developed by an occupational therapist, Jean Ayres, in the 1960s. Ayres focused on the neurological processes that enable the individual to take in and use information from the body and environment to produce organized motor behaviour (Ayres 1972, Fisher and Bundy 1992).

The approach is based on the assumption that learning is dependent on the ability to take in sensory information from the environment (including vestibular, proprioceptive, visual, auditory and tactile data), to process and integrate these sensory inputs within the CNS, and to use this information to plan and produce organized behaviour. Because these processes are fundamental it is suggested that they may affect a wide variety of emotional and behavioural aspects of the child's behaviour as well as the ability to learn academic skills.

SI theory was originally intended to explain mild-to-moderate problems in learning that cannot be attributed to discrete CNS disorders or peripheral sensory loss (Fisher and Bundy 1992). Like the previously described approaches its use has been adapted to children and adults with neurological impairments including CP, and has also been combined with the neurodevelopmental approach to treatment (Blanche 1995). As a significant number of children with CP have sensory impairments, SI may be useful to enable the child to take in and process sensory information better and therefore enhance function. But as the Sensory

Profile of Dunn and Catana (1997) suggests, some children seek and need sensory input because of an inability to register sensory information, whereas others avoid input because of a sensitivity to stimulation. It is not simply a matter of providing more sensory input to those with low registration and desensitizing those who are over-responsive (Dunn and Catana 1997, Dunn 2000).

Lesser known but popular approaches

MOVEMENT OPPORTUNITIES VIA EDUCATION (MOVE)

This 'educational' approach was created in the USA and is prevalent in some areas of the UK. The programme aims to bring sitting, standing and walking opportunities to all with severe disability and offers training and ongoing support to people with disabilities, including parents, carers, and healthcare and other professionals. Education is seen as a means of systematically acquiring motor skills. Equipment (in conjunction with an equipment manufacturer) is used to assist performance and practice of function, *e.g.* eating, toileting, moving from place to place. The aim is to combine therapy with education, a different concept from CE which sees the basis of the whole of the child's behaviour as education.

THE INSTITUTE FOR THE ACHIEVEMENT OF HUMAN POTENTIAL (IAHP)

This institute promoted a programme of intensive sensorimotor therapy based on the philosophy proposed by Glenn Doman and Carl Delacato in Philadelphia, USA (Doman *et al*. 1960). One of the main elements of the intervention is a procedure called 'patterning', which they interpreted to require that the child's whole body is rhythmically moved so as to mimic an amphibian pattern of locomotion. This idea is predicated on an outdated understanding of brain function based on Temple Fay's theory of neurological organization, *i.e.* reflexive behaviour through to recognition and understanding (Temple-Fay 1954), which suggested that brain function becomes increasingly organized during development in a stage-by-stage process from a 'primitive' to a mature state both phylogenetically and ontogenetically. Examples of this are the reflexive response to light (eye blink), progressing through to the ability to read fluently, and crawling with a crossed pattern before walking; in order to develop effectively, each stage must be fully achieved before moving on to the next, *e.g.* a child must crawl before walking. Thus the programme included not only patterned amphibian movement but also 'brachiation' (moving from bar to bar suspended by the arms, as a simian would through trees). This treatment was prescribed to all those with a neurological locomotor impairment or delay, such as CP, without there being any evidence for its efficacy. Typically, children are seen not to need to follow a rigid sequence of development, *e.g.* some children do not crawl but still learn to walk. However, this treatment is not alone within CP therapy in lacking a coherent rationale; what separated it from other modalities was its absolute rigidity which was time consuming, socially demanding and placed considerable stress on the family, because success or failure depended entirely upon them. It was claimed that the system 'worked' and that if their child did not make progress it was because they had not followed the treatment correctly or intensively enough. Rather than working on daily life activities, therapy sessions consist of different activities carried out for about five minutes each during a 30-minute session, with six to eight sessions a day, seven days a week. Sessions are totally organized, indeed regimented might be the right word. The intensity of the programme requires several people 'patterning' (moving the child in precise ways) in unison. Patterning is viewed as a fundamental part of the programme. However, it is passive and not thought to carry over into voluntarily or self-generated activity. Other aspects of the programme include spinning upside-down, suspended from the feet; 'masking' airways so that the child inhales previously expired air (believed to improve brain oxygenation by provoking deeper respiration); brachiation (see above); and an intelligence programme that relies on the use of 'flash cards' which present single pictures or words to the child.

The institute and its methods were at one time strongly promoted and very popular with families who were seeking unconventional therapy, and it was the cause of great concern to paediatric health professionals, particularly in North America. In 1968, a statement openly criticizing the Doman–Delacato method of treatment was published in several journals, which had been approved by many professional bodies in North America, including the American Academy of Paediatrics and the American Academy of Neurology (1967) and the American Academy of Physical Medicine and Rehabilitation (1968).

The Institute for Human Potential took suit against the author and some of the organizations involved, and it took some years for the suit to be dismissed.

In 1988 a further critical discussion of the method was published by Cummins in a full-length book offering a detailed analysis and critiques of the approach, and again the author commented on the problems the programme presented for parents and the lack of any rationale for the treatments.

In 1999 the American Academy of Paediatrics published a review on patterning and concluded that treatment programmes that offer patterning remain unfounded. The treatment is based on oversimplified and outdated theories and there is no robust scientific evidence to support it. Since then further studies have failed to find the intervention successful and none has given these programmes positive endorsement.

BRITISH INSTITUTE FOR BRAIN INJURED CHILDREN; BRAINWAVE
Although originally run in conjunction with the Institute for the Achievement of Human Potential, the Institute's subsequent change of emphasis from treating pathology toward the further improvement of the intellect of the so-called 'gifted children' prompted a split from the parent institute. Thus the British Institute for Brain Injured Children (BIBIC) was conceived. Since then other programmes offering a similar approach have been developed, e.g. 'Brainwave' (also in the UK).

Like the IAHP, the British group uses their own developmental profile, which enables the identification of specific areas of development according to Temple Fay's theory of neurological organization. (Temple-Fay 1954).

Paediatric health professionals within the UK had similar concerns to their North American colleagues, and when reviewed by an independent assessor BIBIC's educational programme was considered to be superficial and did not allow the child to learn comprehension and problem-solving skills (Morton et al. 1997). Play, which is typically a child's primary activity, was notably absent from the programme.

Although BIBIC claim that they no longer follow the Doman–Delacato approach to neurodisability and have modified their programme, an independent review concluded that the underlying influences remained strong (Judge 1999, Morton *et al.* 1999). It was considered that the benefits of the BIBIC programmes are uncertain and that the demands, emotional, financial and other, on the family are considerable (Morton *et al.* 1997).

Approaches that claim to cure

Although the disease process of CP can be modified, the brain damage, although not progressive, is irreparable and there is no cure. However, some groups have claimed to be able to cure or to prevent its occurrence, notably Advance Neuromotor Rehabilitation (ANR). Others, namely Katona and Vojta (see Brandt *et al.* 1980), propose that early signs suggestive of CP in the infant require treatment to avoid the development of CP. However, as we have learnt more about the early development of these so-called at-risk infants, it is quite clear that they would have developed typically with or without treatment. Of more concern are those who directly state that they can change the future of the child with CP from one of chronic disability to predictable step-by-step recovery. This is the claim made by ANR (www.ANR.org.uk).

KATONA

The rationale for the treatment advocated by Katona at the Paediatric Institute Szabadsaghehy, Budapest, is that in infancy the CNS can be modified via a treatment programme. This programme, given six times daily for 30 minutes, is suggested to 'cure' the abnormalities observed to be present following a one-week assessment. However, it is likely that most of the babies treated are mildly affected, and would have developed normally in any case, with or without treatment. As with Vojta (see below), the Katona approach consists of provoking movement patterns from the baby, with the idea that these early patterns are important for CNS connectivity and functional localization. However, Katona recognizes that the early movement patterns are more complex than the simple reflex movements described by Vojta, and are precursors of the later spontaneous activities of posture and locomotion (Katona 1989). The basic patterns also provide a diagnostic tool to detect problems of motor development in the infant, particularly in the first three months of life when such patterns predominate. These patterns also form the basis of the motor training (which must be carried out by the parents for a minimum of three hours per day) and are thought to stimulate central organization of motor control. Thus the emphasis is on motor control, and the statistics that claim that 45% of the CP infants under their programme reached normal motor development may neglect other aspects of development such as sensory, perceptual and cognitive areas, although their importance is acknowledged (Katona 1989). In the same paper it was also accepted that children who were significantly motor impaired require further motor rehabilitation.

VOJTA

The Vojta method (1984) is a well-established therapy intervention in Europe and has some similarities to Katona. While Katona emphasizes the presence of early patterns of sitting, creeping and crawling suggested to be present in the newborn and young infant, Vojta targets what is termed 'reflex locomotion' (this comprises reflex creeping and reflex turning) also considered to be present in utero and at birth (von Aufschnaiter 1992). The Vojta method is primarily considered to be a facilitatory approach that can be applied to all neuromuscular conditions, not just CP.

Vojta views the persistence of these newborn patterns in a child with CP as simply a blocking of postural development, which can be unblocked and activated by facilitating reflex locomotion (Vojta 1984). It is thought that these patterns can then be stored within the nervous system and used spontaneously if the brain has the capacity to do so. Vojta recognized, however, that that there are limits to treatment and that children who are more severely impaired will progress more slowly or may reach the limit of their potential.

Studies to compare Vojta and Bobath have found no significant difference in developmental progress; however, the Vojta approach has been criticized for the emotional stress it may produce on both the child and family (d'Avignon et al. 1981, Ludewig and Mahler 1999).

ADVANCE NEUROMOTOR REHABILITATION

This approach originated in Russia, and although it is not used by many of the CP population it is included here because it is highly controversial and makes dubious claims. These claims cannot be believed and can only serve to mislead and destroy hope in people who are already in a fragile situation. Like BIBIC it demands a rigid approach by the parents, and suggests that three hours per day are required to carry out the regime.

Assessment is done by means of EEG (electrical activity patterns recorded from the brain) and cerebral blood flow measurement. ANR claims to restore the capacity of weak and underdeveloped muscles over which the child with CP has no control.

The programme is physical, metabolic and thermodynamic, i.e. there is direct manipulation of muscles manually, use of hyperbaric oxygen (HBO), provision of amino acids and strengthening of weak muscles. Evaluation of the whole programme is lacking; however, it is known that results of the use of HBO are inconclusive and that no significant benefit has been shown (Collet et al. 2001, Hardy et al. 2002).

Alternative/complementary therapies

Although it is also part of the ANR programme, HBO has emerged as an alternative therapy in its own right in many regions including North America, Europe, India, South Africa and Cuba. There are said to be 64 different conditions, including CP, treated using HBO, although there is only evidence to support its use in 12 of them (Essex 2003). Despite this there are known to be 64 centres for the treatment of multiple sclerosis (MS) with HBO within the UK and Ireland alone (James 2003). Although studies of its efficacy have been carried out (Montgomery et al. 1999; Collet et al. 2001), so far the controls have been inadequate (Essex 2003), and we need more robust scientific evidence to support its use simply because of the reported risks. What these risks are is uncertain as some of them may apply only to the higher pressures (>2 atmospheres) used for divers rather than the lower pressures (≤1.75 atmospheres) used for CP. Nevertheless, even at these lower pressures the risk to hearing has been shown to be real, while the risk to vision (myopia) has not been disproven.

The rationale of HBO treatment is that the amount of oxygen available to the nerve cells will be increased, and this may revive areas of the brain that were deprived of oxygen due to the initial insult. HBO is also considered to reduce brain swelling by the process of blood vessel constriction. While this may well be the case immediately following acute pathologies such as stroke, CP usually results from a lesion either *in utero* or around the time of delivery and is not diagnosed until many months later, so the mechanisms by which HBO may work in acute circumstances may not be relevant.

The treatment requires many sessions—one centre prescribes two sessions per day, five or six days per week for three to four weeks (www.hbotoday.com); another (Collet *et al.* 2001) recommends treatment every weekday for eight weeks, usually at least 40 one-hour sessions. The potential side-effects such as lung damage (pneumothorax) and audio and visual disturbances cannot be dismissed, even if some are rare, and the hazard of the increased risk of igniting flammable materials must also be considered.

There is a long history of how novel treatments for CP have engendered strongly held and opposing views, and the use of HBO is no exception to this pattern. This is a pity because it may make it more difficult to establish whether this is a treatment that has a place within CP. Currently the evidence, like the opinions, backs each extreme. For instance, two of the authors of one study (Collet *et al.* 2001) have stated that the effects of treatment "were statistically and clinically very significant" and that "some children started to walk, to speak, or to sit for the first time in their lives" (Marois and Vanasse 2003). However, the original article also stated that "HBO did not improve the condition of children with cerebral palsy (CP) compared with slightly pressurised air", which would suggest that the specific treatment may not have been the direct cause of any improvement. Similarly with the dangers of HBO: Essex (2003) citing Leach *et al.* (1998) lists the associated hazards, but these are considered not to apply to the lower pressures used for CP treatment (James 2003, Marois and Vanasse 2003), although in one study (Collet *et al.* 2001) over half the children receiving HBO had ear problems.

Therefore, given our current knowledge and the known and possible side-effects, parents should consult their paediatrician before volunteering their child for this treatment, and my own view is that the potential side-effects, though rare, are serious and therefore a decision to try HBO as a treatment for CP must remain questionable. Indeed the summary of a recent review carried out by the Agency for Healthcare Research and Quality (2003) stated that there is insufficient evidence as to whether the use of HBO will improve functional outcomes for children with CP.

Summary
The approach to therapy has changed over the last 100 years from an orthopaedic approach through to a neurophysiological, educational and biomechanical perspective. No one of these approaches alone can provide the answer to the children's and families' needs, but aspects of all are likely to be of some value. Certainly the neurophysiological approaches have neglected the biomechanical and learning factors, as much as the early orthopaedists from

their experience with polio neglected the role of the brain in the organization of movement and function. In a study on goal-oriented reaching, it was concluded that biomechanical factors and neurological processes are complementary to each other for motor planning and ongoing motor control, and as such need to be viewed from that perspective (Martenuik *et al*. 1987). We need to approach management of the child with CP with a balanced viewpoint that is centred on the families' needs and goals, and takes into account the maintenance of muscle length, attention to muscle strength, and the importance of meaningful goals and self-generated activity (Mayston 2001; see also Chapter 11).

In general, families rely on the judgement of professionals to direct them towards appropriate services; however, it must be recognized that access to information via the internet has enabled parents to seek out what they perceive might be useful to them. There are advantages and disadvantages to this—parents can explore the options for themselves and have more choice for their child's future, but some approaches offer more than what is realistically possible and may lure parents into a situation that offers false hope. This often leads them to waste and exhaust their personal resources, financially, emotionally and physically. Cure is not possible; to suggest that it can be provided is irresponsible, and those who do so may be considered to be guilty of misrepresentation. Modification of the condition as it changes over time with growth, experience and development in all areas of ability is possible, but the degree of change will depend largely on the severity of the CP. Whatever management is applied should be seen in these terms, *i.e.* as a modification of the sequelae resulting from the disease process, which will enable the child and family to have the best possible quality of life, despite the severity of the condition.

Conclusion

This chapter has reviewed the main currently applied named approaches to the management of CP (recognizing that these represent only the tip of the iceberg), and it should be clear that no one approach can meet every individual's total needs. Long-held beliefs and myths surrounding therapy need to be examined, and therapy approaches constantly reviewed in the light of current and emerging knowledge. Therapy should be based on the available evidence as far as possible, recognizing that at this moment we do not have enough evidence to base all therapy intervention on experimental evidence, particularly for the child with severe disability and participation restriction. This does not mean that we should discard empirical strategies that seem to work, *e.g.* handling activities that stretch muscles and facilitate movement and function, training functional tasks. What is needed is constant review of therapy strategies in the light of emerging knowledge and evidence, so that families can be offered a treatment that is rational, effective and realistic.

REFERENCES

Agency for Healthcare Research and Quality (2003) 'Hyperbaric oxygen therapy for brain injury, cerebral palsy and stroke.' Department of Health and Human Services, USA: www.ahrq.gov/clinic/tp/hboxtp.htm
American Academy of Pediatrics and American Academy of Neurology (1967) 'Joint executive board statement. Doman–Delacato treatment of neurologically handicapped children.' *Neurology*, **17**, 637.
American Academy of Pediatrics. Committee on Children with Disabilities (1999) 'The treatment of neurologically impaired children using patterning (RE9919).' *Pediatrics*, **104**, 1149–1151.

American Academy of Physical Medicine and Rehabilitation (1968) 'Official statement. The Doman–Delacato treatment of neurologically handicapped children.' *Archives of Physical Medicine and Rehabilitation*, **49**, 183–186.

Ayres, A.J. (1972) *Sensory Integration and Learning Disorders*. Los Angeles: Western Psychological Services.

Bairstow, P., Cochrane, R., Hur, J. (1993) *Evaluation of Conductive Education for Children with Cerebral Palsy*. London: HMSO.

Blanche, E. (1995) 'Cerebral palsy.' *In:* Blanche E, Botticelli T, Holloway M. (Eds.) *Combining Neurodevelopmental and Sensory Integration Principles: An Approach to Physical Therapy*. New York: Psychological Corporation, pp. 67–84.

Bobath, K., Bobath, B. (1984) 'The Neurodevelopmental Treatment.' *In:* Scrutton, D. (Ed.) *Management of the Motor Disorders of Children with Cerebral Palsy. Clinics in Developmental Medicine No. 90*. London: Spastics International Medical Publications, pp. 6–18.

Bower, E., McLellan, D.L. (1994) 'Assessing motor-skill acquisition in four centres for the treatment of children with cerebral palsy.' *Developmental Medicine and Child Neurology*, **36**, 902–909.

Bower, E., McLellan, D.L., Arney, J., Campbell, M.J. (1996) 'A randomised controlled trial of different intensities of physiotherapy and different goal-setting procedures in 44 children with cerebral palsy.' *Developmental Medicine and Child Neurology*, **38**, 226–237.

Bower, E., Michell, D., Burnett, M., Campbell, M.J., McLellan, D.L. (2001) 'Randomized controlled trial of physiotherapy in 56 children with cerebral palsy followed for 18 months.' *Developmental Medicine and Child Neurology*, **43**, 4–15.

Brandt, S., Lonstrup, H.V., Marner, T., Rump, K.J., Selmar, P., Schack, L.K., d'Avignon, M., Noren, L., Arman, T. (1980) 'Prevention of cerebral palsy in motor risk infants by treatment *ad modum* Vojta. A controlled study.' *Acta Paediatrica Scandinavica*, **69**, 283–286.

Butler, C., Darrah, J. (2001) 'Effects of neurodevelopmental treatment (NDT) for cerebral palsy: an AACPDM evidence report.' *Developmental Medicine and Child Neurology*, **43**, 778–790.

Carr, J., Shepherd R. (1998) *Neurological Rehabilitation: Optimizing Motor Performance*. Oxford: Butterworth Heinemann.

Cioni, G. (2002) 'Natural history and treatment of disabilities.' *Developmental Medicine and Child Neurology*, **44**, 651. (Editorial.)

Collet. J.P., Vanasse, M., Marois, P., Amar, M., Goldberg, J., Lambert, J., Lassonde, M., Hardy, P., Fortin, J., Tremblay, S.D., Montgomery, D., Lacroix, J., Robinson, A., Majnemer, A. (2001) 'Hyperbaric oxygen for children with cerebral palsy: a randomised multicentre trial.' *Lancet*, **357**, 582–586.

Cummins, R. (1998) *The Neurologicallyimpaired Child: Doman–Delacato Techniques Reappraised*. New York: Croom Helm.

Damiano, D.L., Abel, M.F. (1998) 'Functional outcomes of strength training in spastic cerebral palsy.' *Archives of Physical Medicine and Rehabilitation*, **79**, 119–125.

d'Avignon, M., Noren, L., Arman, T. (1981) 'Early physiotherapy ad modum Vojta or Bobath in infants with suspected neuromotor disturbance.' *Neuropediatrics*, **12**, 232–241.

Doman, R.J., Spitz, E.R., Zucman, E., Delacato, C.H., Doman, G. (1960) 'Children with severe brain injuries: neurological organization in terms of mobility.' *Journal of the American Medical Association*, **174**, 257–262.

Dunn, W. (2000) 'Sensory issues.' Paper presented at the NDTA Conference, Cincinatti.

Dunn, W., Catana, B. (1997) 'Factor analysis of the sensory profile from a national sample of children without disabilities.' *American Journal of Occupational Therapy*, **51**, 25–34.

Essex, C. (2003) 'Hyperbaric oxygen and cerebral palsy: no proven benefit and potentially harmful.' *Developmental Medicine and Child Neurology*, **45**, 213–215.

Fisher, A.G., Bundy, A.C. (1992) 'Sensory integration therapy.' *In:* Forssberg, H., Hirschfeld, H. (Eds.) *Movement Disorders in Children. Proceedings of the International Sven Jerring Symposium, Stockholm, August 25–29, 1991. Medicine and Sport Science Vol. 36*. Basel: Karger, pp. 16–20.

Flett, P.J. (2003) 'Rehabilitation of spasticity and related problems in childhood cerebral palsy.' *Journal of Paediatrics and Child Health*, **39**, 6–14.

Graves, P. (1995) 'Therapy methods for cerebral palsy.' *Journal of Paediatrics and Child Health*, **31**, 24–28.

Hadders-Algra, M. (2001) 'Early brain damage and the development of motor behavior in children: clues for therapeutic intervention?' *Neural Plasticity*, **8**, 31–49.

Hadders-Algra, M., Brogren, E., Forssberg, H. (1996) 'Training affects the development of postural adjustments in sitting infants.' *Journal of Physiology*, **493**, 289–298.

158

Hardy, P., Collet, J.P., Goldberg, J., Ducruet, T., Vanasse, M., Lambert, J., Marois, P., Amar, M., Montgomery, D.L., Lecomte, J.M., Johnston, K.M. Lassonde, M. (2002) 'Neuropsychological effects of hyperbaric oxygen therapy in cerebral palsy.' *Developmental Medicine and Child Neurology*, **44**, 436–446.

Hari, M., Tillemans, T. (1984) 'Conductive education.' *In:* Scrutton, D. (Ed.) *Management of the Motor Disorders of Children with Cerebral Palsy. Clinics in Developmental Medicine No. 90.* London: Spastics International Medical Publications, pp. 19–35.

Hur, J.J. (1995) 'Review of research on therapeutic interventions for children with cerebral palsy.' *Acta Neurologica Scandinavica*, **91**, 423–432.

Hurvitz, E.A., Leonard, C., Ayyangar, R., Nelson, V.S. (2003) 'Complementary and alternative medicine use in families of children with cerebral palsy.' *Developmental Medicine and Child Neurology*, **45**, 364–370.

James, P. (2003) 'Hyperbaric oxygenation for children with cerebral palsy.' Developmental Medicine and Child Neurology, 45, 648. *(Letter.)*

Judge, J. (1999) 'Multidisciplinary appraisal of the British Institute for Brain Injured Children, Somerset, UK.' *Developmental Medicine and Child Neurology*, **41**, 430. *(Letter.)*

Katona, F. (1989) 'Clinical neurodevelopmental diagnosis and treatment.' *In:* Zelazo, P.R., Barr, R.G. (Eds.) *Challenges to Developmental Paradigms: Implications for Theory, Assessment and Treatment.* London: Lawrence Erlbaum, pp. 167–187.

Knox, V.J., Evans, A.L.E. (2002) 'Evaluation of the functional effects of a course of Bobath therapy in children with cerebral palsy: a preliminary study.' *Developmental Medicine and Child Neurology*, **44**, 447–460.

Leach, R.M., Rees, P.J., Wilmshurst, P. (1998) 'Hyperbaric oxygen therapy.' *British Medical Journal*, **317**, 1140–1143.

Logan, L.R. (2002) 'Facts and myths about therapeutic interventions in cerebral palsy: integrated goal development.' *Physical Medicine and Rehabilitation Clinics of North America*, **13**, 979–989.

Ludewig, A., Mahler, C. (1999) 'Early Vojta- or Bobath-physiotherapy: what is the effect on mother–child relationship?' *Praxis der Kinderpsychologie und Kinderpsychiatrie*, **48**, 326–339.

Marois, P., Vanasse, M. (2003) 'Hyperbaric oxygen therapy and cerebral palsy.' *Developmental Medicine and Child Neurology*, **45**, 646–647. *(Letter.)*

Martenuik, R.G., Mackenzie, C.L., Jeannerod, M., Athenes, S., Dugas, C. (1987) 'Constraints on human arm movement.' *Canadian Journal of Psychology*, **41**, 365–378.

Mayston, M.J. (2001) 'Effects of and perspectives for the treatment of people with cerebral palsy.' *Neural Plasticity*, **8**, 51–69.

Mayston, M.J. (2002) 'Setting the scene.' *In:* Edwards, S. (Ed.) *Neurological Physiotherapy – A Problem-Solving Approach. 2nd Edn.* Edinburgh: Churchill Livingstone, pp. 3–19.

Montgomery, D., Goldberg, J., Amar, M., Lacroix, V., Lecomte, J., Lambert, J., Vanasse, M., Marois, P. (1999) 'Effects of hyperbaric oxygen therapy on children with spastic diplegic cerebral palsy: a pilot project.' *Undersea and Hyperbaric Medicine*, **235**, 235–242.

Morton, R., Benton, S., Bower, E., Carroll-Few, L., Hankinson, J., Lingham, S., Onslow, D., Rhead, S., Wallis, S., Walter A. (1997) *Multidisciplinary Appraisal of the British Institute for Brain Injured Children.* London: Royal College of Paediatrics and Child Health.

Morton, R., Benton, S., Bower, E., Carroll-Few, L., Hankinson, J., Lingham, S., Onslow, D., Rhead, S., Wallis, S., Walter, A. (1999) 'Multidisciplinary appraisal of the British Institute for Brain Injured Children, Somerset, UK.' *Developmental Medicine and Child Neurology*, **41**, 211. (Letter.)

Nelson, K.N., Ellenberg, J.H. (1982) 'Children who outgrow cerebral palsy.' *Pediatrics*, **69**, 529–536.

Palmer, F.B., Shapiro, B.K., Wachtel, R.C., Allen, M.C., Hiller, J.E., Harryman, S.E., Mosher, B.S., Meinert, C.L., Capute, A.J. (1988) 'The effects of physical therapy on cerebral palsy: a controlled trial in infants with spastic diplegia.' *New England Journal of Medicine*, **318**, 803–808.

Prechtl, H.F., Einspieler, C., Cioni, G., Bos, A.F., Ferrari, F., Sontheimer, D. (1997) 'An early marker for neurological deficits after perinatal brain lesions.' *Lancet*, **349**, 1361–1363.

Reddihough, D., King, J., Coleman, G., Catanese, T. (1998) 'Efficacy of programmes based on Conductive Education for young children with cerebral palsy.' *Developmental Medicine and Child Neurology*, **40**, 763–770.

Temple-Fay, T. (1954) Use of pathological and unlocking reflexes in the rehabilitation of spastics.' *American Journal of Physical Medicine*, **33**, 347.

Vojta, V. (1984) 'The basic elements of treatment according to Vojta.' *In:* Scrutton, D. (Ed.) *Management of the Motor Disorders of Children with Cerebral Palsy. Clinics in Developmental Medicine No. 90.* London: Spastics International Medical Publications, pp. 75–85.

159

von Aufschnaiter, D. (1992) 'Vojta: A neurophysiological treatment.' *In:* Forssberg, H., Hirschfeld, H. (Eds) *Movement Disorders in Children. Proceedings of the International Sven Jerring Symposium, Stockholm, August 25–29, 1991. Medicine and Sport Science Vol. 36.* Basel: Karger, pp. 7–15.

Weindling, M. (2000) 'Intervention after brain injury to reduce disability.' *Seminars in Neonatology,* **5,** 53–60.

White, R. (1984) 'Sensory Integrative Therapy for the cerebral palsied child.' *In:* Scrutton, D. (Ed.) *Management of the Motor Disorders of Children with Cerebral Palsy. Clinics in Developmental Medicine No. 90.* London: Spastics International Medical Publications, pp. 86–95.

11
PHYSIOTHERAPY MANAGEMENT IN CEREBRAL PALSY: MOVING BEYOND PHILOSOPHIES

Diane Damiano

People interact with their world through movement. Physiotherapists train to be 'movement experts'; and patients and other health professionals rely on them for this expertise when movement is disrupted by injury or disease. This is an awesome responsibility that is perhaps even greater for those who have the privilege of working with children. Best medical practice in physiotherapy, as in any field, requires the support of scientific knowledge to the extent that it is available. This is as true and important for treating chronic motor disorders as it is for treating life-threatening illness. The evidence for physical therapy treatment in children with motor disorders has been increasing exponentially in the past several years. Consequently our reliance on philosophical approaches is no longer necessary and may in fact be counter-productive to optimal management.

Top-down versus bottom-up approach
For decades, physiotherapy management of children with cerebral palsy (CP) has been dominated by a top-down philosophical approach. While some philosophies still have a pervasive local or international influence, a gradual but definite paradigm shift has infiltrated the field in the past decade supporting a 'bottom-up' approach that is based less on treatment 'philosophies' and more on treatment 'principles'. In this scenario, treatment recommendations originate from, and are continually modified by, a foundation of basic and clinical scientific principles. This shift is mirrored in the design of this second edition, as compared to the first in which individual chapters were dedicated to the various prevailing philosophies for managing a child with CP. While some of these philosophies have retained a strong presence and following, and new ones have emerged, no one approach has yet been shown to be more effective or advantageous than another, and many clinicians now profess to use a combined or 'eclectic' approach by selecting among these and retaining some components as treatment options, in conjunction with other new treatment strategies that have emerged.

In my view, the time has come for a more radical change in our profession: we need to go a step further and eliminate the adherence to philosophies altogether. Persisting in any philosophy whose basis has uncertain scientific validity or which has been modified so that it no longer resembles the original philosophy or may now signify different things to different people is damaging not only to our profession but, more importantly, to the children we treat. Philosophical adherence may also impede the timely incorporation of scientific evidence into our field and diminish effective intra- and interdisciplinary interaction and respect.

Another potential 'danger' with philosophies is their packaged approach where you either accept or reject the whole package. The adoption of a specific philosophy may lead, intentionally or not, to the rejection of other competing philosophies regardless of their merit, not dissimilar to the choice of a religious faith or a political party. Some may argue that partial acceptance of philosophies is possible and permissible, and this 'eclectic' approach has appealed to many. Philosophies typically incorporate several different treatment strategies of which some are likely to be effective and some not; however, these should be differentiated through scientific study, not selected or rejected based on individual preferences. Ineffective strategies should be deleted from the 'menu', and effective strategies should be retained, but removed from under their philosophical 'umbrella'.

Philosophies vary in the degree to which they are tolerant or intolerant of other approaches, and in some instances, success or failure of a philosophical approach has been attributed to how faithful the user, whether therapist or family and patient, was to that philosophy. While some philosophies are rigid in their application even in the face of contradictory evidence, others are open to and accepting of change leading to a new dilemma of at what point does it become a different philosophy that would no longer be recognizable or true to its originator?

On a more positive side, philosophies do provide a coherent and systematic approach to treatment that has much appeal to clinicians and families (Scrutton 1984). However, a strong scientific basis for treatment, if sufficiently large and well formulated, should be able to provide a similar if not higher level of assurance.

Evidence-based treatment principles in cerebral palsy

Scientific evidence for treatments addressing motor dysfunction in persons with CP and other neuromotor disorders is continually and rapidly accumulating. Treatment rationales, clinical assumptions and existing interventions are being evaluated more closely, and novel therapies are under investigation as well. While more evidence is becoming available, much work remains. Relatively few randomized clinical trials have been published in these areas, not all treatments have been subjected to equally rigorous investigation, evidence on relative effectiveness among treatment options is scarce, and additional parameters such as timing and intensity of interventions have yet to be well-defined. While the state of the evidence shows many deficiencies, enough scientific support is now available to suggest that our previous approaches warrant serious reconsideration (Butler and Darrah 2001).

The cerebral palsies are now recognized as a collection of disorders, the common unifying feature of which is a defect or injury to an immature nervous system that adversely affects motor coordination. The motor disability may range from negligible to severe, and regardless of degree, may coexist with or be eclipsed by other chronic or acute abnormalities in an individual patient. Ideally, treatment of the motor disorder is multidisciplinary, involving a partnership among the patient and family, health professionals and the community to optimize functional mobility and health-related quality of life for each individual. Physiotherapists may provide direct treatment as part of an overall management plan based on specific patient goals or may serve a more consultative role. Regardless of discipline, role of the team or clinical setting, treatment recommendations should be developed based on current scientific evidence or, in the absence of evidence, be consistent with current scientific principles. Novel or untested therapies, particularly those that defy existing physiological principles, should be treated with scepticism until supportive evidence can be provided.

Specific strategies for management of the motor disorder will be discussed below, recognizing that due to the dynamic nature of scientific knowledge, some of these may be outdated or warrant revision even by the time this book is in press. Each will be grouped and then discussed within the context of one of five potential therapeutic aims when working with a patient with a chronic motor disorder as listed below:

1. to reduce current musculoskeletal impairments so as to improve function and quality of life in the short and long term
2. to enable children to function optimally given their existing impairments
3. to prevent or limit development of secondary impairments that may further limit function
4. to alter the 'natural' course of the disorder
5. to promote wellness and fitness over the lifespan.

REDUCING CURRENT MUSCULOSKELETAL IMPAIRMENTS SO AS TO IMPROVE FUNCTION AND QUALITY OF LIFE

After a patient, parents and clinical team identify a functional goal, detailed assessment will help to ascertain which impairments are limiting the ability to achieve that goal, and then a multidisciplinary treatment plan, of which therapy is an integral part, is devised that will address those impairments and progress towards that functional goal.

For example, a pre-adolescent girl with a diagnosis of spastic diplegia states that her goal is to be able to walk longer distances in a faster, more continuous manner so that she could attend her new school without a wheelchair. At the present time, she is unable to take more than 20 steps before needing to rest. Assessment revealed a very slow, laborious gait pattern with severe crouch at the hips, knees and ankles throughout the gait cycle. Steps lengths were very short, and her trunk and upper extremities moved excessively to generate momentum for advancing her legs. She has orthoses, but insists that they are too uncomfortable, and she does not use any assistive devices despite her frequent falls and increasing need to catch or stabilize herself on nearby objects.

For this hypothetical patient, many factors may be disrupting her ability to take multiple continuous steps. After determining which one(s) are limiting her desired goal to the greatest extent, some type of direct treatment would typically be recommended to address one or more musculoskeletal or neurological impairments, which may include restricted muscle length, spasticity, weakness, poor cardiovascular fitness or pain, among others. Depending on the primary factors involved, medication, surgery, an exercise programme, new orthotics, a hand-held assistive device for walking, or any combination of the above, may be warranted.

The physiotherapy programme would potentially focus on augmenting the lengthening effects of orthopaedic surgery, spasticity reduction, or botulinum toxin injections through stretching, casting, increased activity and patient education. Day and/or nighttime use of ankle orthoses could also aid in this goal. Strengthening the muscles that provide support of the body during upright postures and/or those that accelerate the body through space and allow the foot to clear the ground may be needed. To gain strength, a muscle must be loaded at a high percentage of its maximum voluntary force. Free weights, exercise devices, electrical stimulation or manual resistance are modalities that can be used to induce muscle strength changes. Multiple studies have now been published in CP demonstrating the effectiveness of several types of strengthening programmes (see reviews by Damiano *et al.* 2002, Dodd *et al.* 2002).

Treadmill training has been shown to increase strength, gait speed, step symmetry, co-ordination of reciprocal activity, and/or endurance, and may also be included as a component of an exercise programme. The exact parameters of treadmill use such as amount of weight support (if any), the belt speed and duration of walking can be adjusted to accomplish specific goals. The physiological effects of treadmill training have been well documented in the literature in other populations. Evidence on the benefits unique to rehabilitation has been accumulating in recent years with reports showing improved gait symmetry and speed, positive changes in ambulatory status, and improvement in generalized gross motor function (Schindl *et al.* 2000). Physical activities outside of therapy or participation in sports should also be encouraged whenever possible to increase strength and endurance as well as to promote other physical, emotional and social benefits. Overground gait training may also be implemented, and specific coordination patterns may be practiced to improve gait quality, efficiency and adaptability.

ENABLING PEOPLE TO FUNCTION OPTIMALLY GIVEN THEIR EXISTING IMPAIRMENTS
This category may include direct interventions to help patients solve motor problems, that is to learn and practice new functional movement strategies to compensate for motor abilities that were lost or have not yet developed. This aim assumes that any existing impairments that interfered with movement were already addressed to the maximum extent possible or desired. 'Normal' movement or approximating that may not necessarily be the goal. What is important is that the movement pattern being learned optimizes function and participation in the short term without potential interference on future goals or adverse effects on the musculoskeletal system in the long term. Unfortunately, data on the long-term results of our treatment strategies are not readily available so we may not know for certain whether we are sacrificing long-term function for short-term goals. Our knowledge of physiology and biomechanics should guide us to prefer strategies that are more likely to preserve muscle length and power, that minimize abnormal loads on joints that could lead to pain and deformity, and that restrict mobility to the least extent possible.

The therapist may also need to be assisting the patient and family in making equipment decisions to enhance mobility and participation. The old dogma that providing powered mobility or augmentative communication devices will limit the further development of independent walking or speech skills has been shown to be untrue (Butler 1986). Technological advances continue to increase the options for independence and functional enhancement in persons with disabilities, and our awareness, local availability and expense are often the greatest limitations to their incorporation.

What is less often considered in physical therapy is the potential adverse effect of not doing something, or not doing it soon enough or aggressively enough. Basic scientific evidence on the effects of immobilization on the musculoskeletal system has been reported by several authors (Goldspink *et al.* 1995, Gajdosik and Cicirello 2001). For example, by not encouraging more physical activity in patients who have challenges in their abilities to move, muscle tightness and weakness may be exacerbated. Over time, the muscle fibres themselves may change histologically or fail to grow normally (Booth *et al.* 2001). Based on Wolfe's Law, bones may develop insufficiently or abnormally due to inappropriate muscle activity or altered loading patterns. The development of motor coordination is impeded by a reduction in the amount and variety of movement experiences. Therapists are often in a position of playing 'catch-up' by trying to alleviate the impairments that eventually develop; however, a more satisfactory solution may be greater prevention of this process by encouraging more and earlier activity.

While muscle cells are not mature at birth and the process of myelination of pathways is not complete, the peripheral musculoskeletal system has the capacity to be normal prior to the brain lesion. In infancy an overabundance of cortical pathways has been noted, and the fate of these is use-dependent (Eyre *et al.* 2001). With diminished or inappropriate use, the development of muscles, bones and the brain is compromised, often permanently. Not all muscles are similarly affected; therefore, disruptions in the physiological balance of muscle forces across joints occur that can lead to or exacerbate deformity. Therapists must be alert to the issue of 'relative' as well as 'absolute' muscle strength when conducting strengthening programmes. Recent evidence also suggests that weakness of a muscle may contribute to the development of muscle shortening (Shortland *et al.* 2002), and strengthening of a muscle may therefore help to maintain its length as well as increase its force-generating capacity. The repeated stretching of the antagonist is also of obvious benefit since muscles must be in their maximally stretched position for at least six hours so as not to lose length (Tardieu *et al.* 1988). Spasticity is often targeted as the primary culprit in restricting muscle length, but diminished selective control, weakness, persistent postures and inactivity must also be considered as potential 'suspects' and addressed proactively.

While early motor intervention seems inherently well justified from a neurophysiological, biomechanical and cognitive perspective, the level of scientific support for this practice is surprisingly unimpressive. Determining the type of programme that should be administered and the most appropriate infants to target are still important research questions. However, it is generally accepted that motor activity should be encouraged and promoted beginning in infancy and preferred whenever possible over static positioning that would serve to maintain muscle length to the same degree, but without the additional benefits that activity provides. For example, a weight-supported walking device (with or without orthoses) that provides only as much body support as needed to maintain optimal biomechanical alignment in the upright position and allows at least some mobility within the home or classroom may be far more preferable than a rigid standing frame. Physical assistance, equipment or environmental manipulations may be needed to facilitate movement opportunities. As the child matures and develops these may be altered in type, intensity and frequency, and adjusted so that they are developmentally appropriate, but moving for the sake of moving is still a laudable goal for physical, social and emotional health.

ALTERING THE 'NATURAL' COURSE OF THE DISORDER

As therapists, we work with patients who have already sustained an injury, or have acquired or been born with a disorder. The natural course of a disorder is considered the expected sequela if no treatments are administered. The natural history of CP in the absence of treatment might be discernible if one were to visit an underdeveloped country with few medical resources, but has been well disguised from most of us by our interventions. However, some expected patterns of change have been detected within the current 'standard of care' (Rodda and Graham 2001, Rosenbaum *et al.* 2002). Rang and Wright (1989) made the astute and humbling observation years ago that we can clearly make people with CP different, but we cannot be so certain that they are better. All children, including those with CP, typically undergo rapid change in the early years, and motor coordination continues to develop well into the teen years (Damiano and Abel 2002, Rosenbaum *et al.* 2002). Therefore, we cannot necessarily attribute all positive changes that occur to our interventions. Instead we need to show that our interventions have exceeded the expected rates of change or have minimized or prevented the expected progression of deformity. Regression equations (Rosenbaum *et al.* 2002) have been developed that can estimate expected improvement in gross motor performance in CP over time as a function of age and current motor abilities. Randomized trials can provide definitive evidence regarding the type and amount of change that can be attributed to interventions alone; however, ethical issues of withholding treatment or random assignment to high-risk treatments are difficult to surmount.

The fact that CP occurs before the central and peripheral nervous systems fully develop and mature is a source of both optimism and pessimism. Optimistically, we can hope to reap some benefits from and perhaps even further facilitate the inherent plasticity of an infant and toddler's brain. Pessimistically, we are concerned about the developmental 'pruning' process of potential or existing pathways that are not being utilized that may further limit prognosis, and the secondary effects of brain abnormalities on the development of the musculoskeletal system. Recent advances in neuroscience suggest the exciting possibility that consistent and fairly intense patterned motor activity may have neural regenerative effects on the damaged nervous system (McDonald *et al.* 2002); however, much work needs to be done before we can apply this to chronic models of brain injury particularly in animals whose recoveries may be confounded by developmental events. Imaging studies have shown changes in the damaged sensorimotor cortex of brain-injured adults and children that correlate with functional gains as a result of interventions such as constraint-induced therapy and botulinum toxin injections (Boyd *et al.* 2002, Taub *et al.* 2002). Cognitive learning theories have provided insights on the type and intensity of practice that facilitates the learning of new skills, including motor tasks, that are being incorporated into therapy strategies for facilitating motor learning and control in normal and damaged nervous systems (see Chapter 6). Findings such as these may revolutionize the role of physical therapy in neurorehabilitation and hopefully provide dramatic alterations in the 'natural' history of brain injuries.

The health benefits of good nutrition and regular exercise across the lifespan are apparent for all individuals, yet disparities in health promotion efforts and opportunities for and accessibility of exercise programmes in the disabled population are known to exist (Rimmer and Damiano 2002). Nutritional interventions are strongly recommended for children with CP who are significantly below normal on standard paediatric growth charts (Samson-Fang *et al*. 2002). The projected benefits include reduced numbers of illnesses, better ability to recover from surgery, and better muscle and bone development, among others. It is also important that physiotherapists advocate for exercise and fitness programmes, and work with patients to help them identify and gain access to available programmes. Therapists can also help patients to develop specific motor skills to augment their participation in regular exercise or sports programmes or recreational activities. Physiotherapists should ideally be in the forefront of encouraging medical delivery systems to be more proactive in supporting wellness as a preventive health practice. Fitness goals should be encouraged as a part of or as an adjunct to therapy, and incorporated into transition plans from therapy. Therapists have ideal backgrounds for working with community resources and programmes to make these more available, safe, sufficiently challenging and rewarding. Examples of programmes with documented effectiveness in CP are aquatic exercise (Peganoff 1984) and horseback riding (Sterba *et al*. 2002), but the list should be much longer and more varied to satisfy different ages, skill levels and interests.

The present and future

New knowledge regarding the cascades of events that can lead to the development of the cerebral palsies (Nelson and Willoughby 2002) and advances in brain imaging (Krageloh-Mann *et al*. 1999) are leading to new preventative strategies and greater diagnostic precision in this population. Although a cure for these disorders once they occur remains elusive, novel treatments are continually emerging that demonstrate promise for brighter functional prognoses. Viable physiotherapy treatment options have expanded in recent years to include muscle strengthening techniques (Damiano *et al*. 2002); repetitive motor training of upper- and lower-extremity skills (Butefisch *et al*. 1995, Hesse *et al*. 2000); task-related training (Dean and Shepherd 1997); constraint-induced therapy for improving upper-extremity use (Taub *et al*. 2002), the basis of which is massed practice of sequentially more challenging functionally relevant tasks; sensorimotor retraining techniques and many others. The use of computerized technology and functional electrical stimulation (Wright and Granat 2000) for facilitating motor rehabilitation are also being actively and creatively explored. New advances in neurorehabilitation suggest that we have not yet maximized the processes of development, plasticity and neural regeneration in patients with motor disorders that could further enhance existing expectations for functional recovery in CP and other central nervous system disorders (McDonald *et al*. 2002). It is possible that permanent destructive surgical techniques may become less favoured as prevention, habilitation and regeneration are optimized.

Summary

Incorporation of principles into physiotherapy practice implies that a scientific rationale

167

for treatment exists and that some level of experimental evidence is available demonstrating that a specific treatment is effective or more ideally efficacious. Some very important and innovative philosophies provided a rationale for treatment prior to the availability of evidence, but these should now be relegated to their rightful place in history. Any old or new philosophical programmes that offer a 'total' approach to therapy that is not based on sound scientific principles, even in part, or fails to allow for the incorporation of other treatments that have been shown to be equally or more effective should be discouraged. I am convinced that sufficient research evidence, much of which has been contributed by physiotherapists themselves, now exists to guide treatments to the extent that philosophical adherence is no longer needed or warranted. The rehabilitation field is experiencing explosive scientific growth, so we also need to remain continually alert to clinical and basic scientific advances in the fields of muscle physiology, neuroscience, biomechanics, cognitive psychology and exercise physiology, among others, for the emergence of new strategies. It is our responsibility as therapists to offer the children that we treat the best that science has to offer them, so they can enjoy and participate in life to the fullest.

REFERENCES

Booth, C.M., Cortina-Boria, M.J., Theologis, T.N. (2001) 'Collagen accumulation in muscles of children with cerebral palsy and correlation with severity of spasticity.' *Developmental Medicine and Child Neurology*, **43**, 314–320.

Boyd, R., Bach, T., Morris, M., Imms, C., Johnson, L., Graham, H.K., Syngeniotis, A., Abbott, D., Jackson, G. (2002) 'A randomized trial of botulinum toxin A and upper limb training—a functional MRI study.' *Developmental Medicine and Child Neurology*, **44**, Suppl. 91, 9. *(Abstract.)*

Butefisch, C., Hummelsheim, H., Denzler, P., Mauritz, K.H. (1995) 'Repetitive training of isolated movements improves the outcome of motor rehabilitation of the centrally paretic hand.' *Journal of the Neurological Scences*, **130**, 59–68.

Butler, C. (1986) 'Effects of powered mobility on self-initiated behaviors of very young children with loco-motor disability.' *Developmental Medicine and Child Neurology*, **28**, 325–332.

Butler, C., Darrah, J. (2001) 'Effects of neurodevelopmental treatment (NDT) for cerebral palsy: an AACPDM evidence report.' *Developmental Medicine and Child Neurology*, **43**, 778–790.

Damiano, D.L., Abel, M.F. (2002) 'Relationships among impairments, motor function, and perceived health status in spastic cerebral palsy: a multi-center collaboration.' *Developmental Medicine and Child Neurology*, **42**, Suppl. 83, 42. *(Abstract.)*

Damiano, D.L., Dodd, K., Taylor, N.F. (2002) 'Should we be testing and training muscle strength in cerebral palsy?' *Developmental Medicine and Child Neurology*, **44**, 68–72.

Dean, C.M., Shepherd, R.B. (1997) 'Task-related training improves performance of seated reaching tasks after stroke. A randomized controlled trial.' *Stroke*, **28**, 722–728.

Dodd, K.J., Taylor, N.F., Damiano, D.L. (2002) 'A systematic review of the effectiveness of strength-training programs for people with cerebral palsy.' *Archives of Physical Medicine and Rehabilitation*, **83**, 1157–1164.

Eyre, J.A., Taylor, J.P., Villagra, F., Smith, M., Miller, S. (2001) 'Evidence of activity-dependent withdrawal of corticospinal projections during human development.' *Neurology*, **57**, 1543–1554.

Gajdosik, C.G., Cicirello, N. (2001) 'Secondary conditions of the musculoskeletal system in adolescents and adults with cerebral palsy.' *Physical and Occupational Therapy in Pediatrics*, **21**, 49–68.

Goldspink, D.F., Cox, V.M., Smith, S.K., Eaves, L.A., Osbaldeston, N.J., Lee, D.M., Mantle, D. (1995) 'Muscle growth in response to mechanical stimuli.' *American Journal of Physiology*, **268**, E288–E297.

Hesse, S., Uhlenbrock, D., Werner, C., Bardeleben, A. (2000) 'A mechanized gait trainer for restoring gait in nonambulatory subjects.' *Archives of Physical Medicine and Rehabilitation*, **81**, 1158–1161.

Krageloh-Mann, I., Toft, P., Lunding, J., Andresen, J., Pryds, O., Lou, H.C. (1999) 'Brain lesions in preterms: origin, consequences and compensation.' *Acta Paediatrica*, **88**, 897–908.

McDonald, J.W., Becker, D., Sadowsky, C.L., Jane, J.A., Conturo, T.E. (2002) 'Late recovery following spinal cord injury. Case report and review of the literature.' *Journal of Neurosurgery*, **97** (Suppl.), 252–265.

Nelson, K.B., Wiloughby, R.E. (2002) 'Overview: infection during pregnancy and neurologic outcome in the child.' *Mental Retardation and Developmental Disabilities Research Reviews*, **8**, 1–2.

Peganoff, S.A. (1984) 'The use of aquatics with cerebral palsied adolescents.' *American Journal of Occupational Therapy*, **38**, 469–473.

Rang, M., Wright, J. (1989) 'What have 30 years of medical progress done for cerebral palsy?' *Clinical Orthopaedics*, **247**, 55–60.

Rimmer, J., Damiano, D.L. (2002) 'Maintaining or improving fitness in children with disabilities.' *In:* Damiano, D.L. (Ed.) *Topics in Physical Therapy – Pediatrics*. Alexandria, VA: American Physical Therapy Association, pp. 1–16.

Rodda, J., Graham, H.K. (2001) 'Classification of gait patterns in spastic hemiplegia and spastic diplegia: a basis for a management algorithm.' *European Journal of Neurology*, **8**, Suppl, 5, 98–108.

Rosenbaum, P.L., Walter, S.D., Hanna, S.E., Palisano, R.J., Russell, D.J., Wood, E., Dartlett, D.J., Galuppi, B.E. (2002) 'Prognosis for gross motor function in cerebral palsy: creation of motor development curves.' *Journal of the American Medical Association*, **288**, 1357–1363.

Samson-Fang, L., Fung, E., Stallings, V.A., Conaway, M., Worley, G., Rosenbaum, P., Calvert, R., O'Donnell, M., Henderson, R.C., Chumlea, W.C., Liptak, G.S., Stevenson, R.D. (2002) 'Relationship of nutritional status to health and societal participation in children with cerebral palsy.' *Journal of Pediatrics*, **141**, 637–643.

Schindl, M.R., Forstner, C., Kern, H., Hesse, S. (2000) 'Treadmill training with partial body weight support in nonambulatory patients with cerebral palsy.' *Archives of Physical Medicine and Rehabilitation*, **81**, 301–306.

Scrutton, D. (Ed.) (1984) *Management of the Motor Disorders of Children with Cerebral Palsy. Clinics in Developmental Medicine No. 90*. London: Spastics International Medical Publications.

Shortland, A.P., Harris, C.A., Gough, M., Robinson, R.O. (2002) 'Architecture of the medial gastrocnemius in children with spastic diplegia.' *Developmental Medicine and Child Neurology*, **44**, 158–163.

Sterba, J.A., Rogers, B.T., France, A.P., Vokes, D.A. (2002) 'Horseback riding in children with cerebral palsy: effect on gross motor function.' *Developmental Medicine and Child Neurology*, **44**, 301–308.

Tardieu, C., Lespargot, A., Tabary, C., Bret, M.D. (1988) 'For how long must the soleus muscle be stretched each day to prevent contracture?' *Developmental Medicine and Child Neurology*, **30**, 3–10.

Taub, E., Uswatte, G., Elbert, T. (2002) 'New treatments in neurorehabilitation founded on basic research.' *Nature Reviews. Neuroscience*, **3**, 228–236.

Wright, P.A., Granat, M.H. (2000) 'Therapeutic effects of functional electrical stimulation of the upper limb of eight children with cerebral palsy.' *Developmental Medicine and Child Neurology*, **42**, 724–727.

169

12
CEREBRAL PALSY IN ADULT LIFE

Susan Edwards

Cerebral palsy (CP) is a life-long condition and yet, whilst there is extensive literature covering aspects of management and treatment of children with CP, there is a relatively little describing the transition into adulthood and beyond.

What happens to individuals with CP when they enter the adult world? Most therapists working in the paediatric field would have several children with CP as part of their caseload. Why therefore is it a rare event for an adult with CP to find their way onto the books of therapists working with adults with neurological disability or musculoskeletal impairments?

CP is defined as being a non-progressive disorder of the brain. This has led to the assumption that the disabilities and handicaps arising from this impairment are also non-progressive but this is clearly not the case (Pimm 1992a). Function and ability change, and it is therefore essential that individuals with CP, and all those involved in their care, recognize how tenuous is their hold on optimal physical performance. Deterioration in the physical condition in such people, even in those with stable pathologies, is inevitable without appropriate intervention (Pope 1997).

Amelioration of the primary condition, cerebral palsy, should not be the focus of health care intervention (Gajdosik and Cicirello 2001). Mayston (2001) suggested that the main aim of therapy for the child with CP should be to improve the quality of life for the individual person and their family and to prepare for improved quality of life during adult years. To this end, three general aims were identified: (1) to increase or improve the skill repertoire, (2) to maintain functional level, and (3) to establish a general management programme to minimize the development of contractures and deformities.

Why should these aims be any different when the child becomes an adult? Surely it is still imperative to maintain the individual's level of achievement and to prevent secondary complications, and yet the importance of consistent attention to maintaining health and function is often not recognized by either the individuals with CP or their health-care providers. Both young adults with CP and their carers expect the condition to remain static and are therefore generally unprepared for the reduced level of function that so often arises as the child becomes an adult (Pimm 1992a, Gajdosik and Cicirello 2001).

What mechanisms are in place for provision of ongoing management and support for this client group? Rehabilitation care with regard to the physical status of adults with CP has been described as being "at best inconsistent" (Murphy *et al.* 1995). This is in spite of the reported incidence of secondary conditions that give rise to a loss of function and deterioration in quality of life (Pimm 1992b, Ando and Ueda 2000, Bottos *et al.* 2001, Gajdosik and Cicirello 2001). Bax *et al.* (1988) interviewed 104 young adults with physical disability, 45 of whom had CP, who reported that their physical condition deteriorated after they had left school; they became less mobile and their contractures more fixed. They said that they had not been reviewed since leaving school, and changes in their motor performance had not been assessed.

There appears to be an almost total lack of any coordinated services for young adults comparable with those put in place by community paediatricians for children (Chamberlain 1993), and those that are available have been described as unfocused and fragmented (Stevenson *et al*. 1997). Although acute illnesses are generally addressed, there is a lack of preventative medicine (Murphy *et al*. 1995) and this lack of service provision for the adult population would seem to put them at greater risk of increasing disablement across their life span (Murphy 1999).

It is also important to appreciate that at the same time as the child enters adolescence and subsequently becomes an adult, so their parents age and have increasing difficulty caring for their disabled child whose stature and weight increases (Pimm 1996, Rapp and Torres 2000, Fiorentino *et al*. 1998). However, whereas the care staff can refuse to handle a client without appropriate provision of manual handling equipment, all too often the parents have no option and may get to the point of breakdown before help is provided.

Against this background, the purpose of this chapter is to identify the problems often encountered by adolescents and adults with CP and to discuss the implications of ongoing management to improve the quality of life for this client group.

Compensatory movement strategies

Children with movement dysfunction will develop various compensatory strategies to enable them to function. However, whilst these strategies may be effective during their early years, over time the abnormal biomechanical forces and immobility often lead to excessive physical stress and strain, overuse syndromes, fatigue and possibly early joint degeneration (Murphy *et al*. 1995, Gajdosik and Cicirello 2001). An illustration of this potential decrease in functional ability is the progressive difficulties encountered with gait. The movement patterns adopted to enable ambulation may lead to lumbar spine and lower limb joint degeneration (Harada *et al*. 1993) and the energy expended in maintaining gait may become unsustainable in later life (Bottos *et al*. 2001, Andersson and Mattsson 2001). Therefore, whilst the use of compensatory patterns of movement is inevitable, promotion of independence skills, particularly walking may need to be tempered. Short-term gains may be offset by the longer-term consequences of premature loss of functional ability (Pimm 1992a).

In a study carried out by Murphy *et al*. (1995), 101 adults with CP were investigated, of whom 49 were described as having spasticity and 52 dyskinesia. Their general health was reported to be similar to an age-matched able-bodied population with the exception of the incidence of urinary tract infection. Fifty-seven subjects had undergone a total of 191 orthopaedic procedures. Sixty-seven were in wheelchairs, 26 of whom had walked previously. Seventy-five per cent of those who had stopped walking had done so by age 25 for reasons of fatigue and inefficiency of gait, with some reporting that wheelchair mobility enabled better function. A second peak occurred at 45 years when people reported that they stopped walking due to painful joints, particularly in the hips, knees and metatarsal heads.

171

Not only do compensatory strategies potentially lead to a gradual loss of function and reduced level of independence but pathological movement patterns may also prevent normal skeletal development and lead to joint derangement. For example, in children with CP, the hips are usually normal at birth, but with growth a combination of muscle imbalance and bony deformity may lead to progressive dysplasia (Flynn and Miller 2002).

Lack of monitoring of progressive secondary conditions such as subluxation or those arising as a result of repetitive movements may result in worsening of the condition until pain or loss of function brings the individual to seek medical attention. Unfortunately, once young adults with CP leave secondary education, they are less likely to see specialists unless they have an acute episode that may at least bring them into contact with the existing services (Bax *et al*. 1988, Condie 1991, Murphy *et al*. 1995, Gajdosik and Cicirello 2001).

Use of aids, adaptive equipment and assistive technology

Compensatory movement strategies also include the use of aids, adaptive equipment and assistive technology, and the maintenance of independence may be determined by their appropriate usage (Williams and Bowie 1993). However, to ensure effective use, it is essential to monitor the changing physical status of the individual with regard to their equipment needs, to appreciate that these needs change as they get older, and to know what is on the market (Gajdosik and Cicirello 2001).

All too often, when assessing the adult population with CP, the equipment that had been supplied had broken over time, or was outmoded, outgrown or inappropriate. Of 78 people with moderate to severe dysarthria, only two had augmentative communication devices, and of the crutches and sticks used, 90% were in a state of disrepair (Murphy *et al*. 1995). This is in stark contrast to the more routine availability of aids and equipment for children with CP (Murphy 1999).

Secondary conditions

Adolescents and adults with CP are routinely affected by secondary complications resulting from their primary impairment. From a physical perspective these include reduced muscle strength and cardiovascular endurance or physiological burn-out (Pimm 1992a), contractures, pain, osteoporosis, increased severity of pathological movement patterns and, in the athetoid population, cervical spondylotic myelopathy (Fuji *et al*. 1987, Darrah *et al*. 1999, Gajdosik and Cicirello 2001). Women with CP also report bladder and bowel problems, and increased spasticity and incontinence during menstruation (Turk *et al*. 2001).

In addition to these physical impairments, social problems have also been identified relating to their activities of daily living, further education, work, acceptance within society, maintaining relationships, sexuality and difficulties with communication. Even those with a high level of independence with regard to mobility, carrying out their functional tasks and with communication, were found to be poorly integrated socially (van der Dussen *et al*. 2001). Not surprisingly, age and progression of disability were found to be important factors when assessing the subjective well-being of people with CP (Furukawa *et al*. 2001).

One of the major difficulties facing adults with CP is that frequently any deterioration in function is attributed to the primary diagnosis (Murphy *et al*. 1995). Communication difficulties and cognitive impairment may make assessment and management of these secondary conditions challenging but this cannot excuse an inadequate medical or therapy examination wherein changing pathology and reduced physical ability is not noticed. While the normal ageing process will inevitably affect function, in adults with CP this is compounded by the existing level of disability (Turk *et al*. 2001).

Reduced muscle strength and cardiovascular endurance (physiological burn-out)

The term physiological burn-out, coined by Pimm (1992b), is an apt description for the gradual loss of function encountered by many adults with CP. It is hypothesized that physiological burn-out is a condition in which motor function declines in relation to the physical demands imposed on the physiological systems. The greater the demands the more likely that physiological burn-out will take place.

The condition is characterized by reduced physical strength, loss of or significant deterioration in mobility and dexterity, deterioration in speech (if the individual has dysarthria) and physical exhaustion. It is suggested that the most vulnerable individuals are those high achievers who strive to improve performance and maximize independence, without recognition of the toll this takes physically. Those who are in paid employment and self-supporting in the home may be most prone to this condition (Pimm 1992b).

Physiological burn-out occurs when prolonged stress is placed on the motor system that is already operating at maximum capacity as a consequence of CP and it is manifested by a gradual and premature loss of functional skills. This deterioration may not be reversible but it is suggested that, with good management and conservation of function, its effects may be delayed or halted (Pimm 1992b). Obviously, a key priority is the acceptance and recognition by health-care professionals of the potential for decline in function, if the clients are expected to function at their maximum level all the time.

Contractures

Contractures are among the most common secondary impairments associated with CP (Cadenhead *et al*. 2002). Their prevention, or at least minimization, is crucial to maintaining the optimum level of function for adults with CP.

Are contractures unavoidable? Although Cadenhead *et al*. (2002) reported that passive exercises were ineffective in preventing contractures, this was based on a study of six adults with CP, all with learning difficulties. One could argue that passive exercise *per se* is unlikely to be effective given that six hours of constant stretch is required to maintain range in a spastic muscle (in this case the soleus muscle) (Tardieu *et al*. 1988). Perhaps the continuation of a regular management programme, usually available to children with CP is required to maintain range of movement. Standing, appropriate seating and positioning in bed, in addition to specific therapy as required would be key features of such a management programme.

Unfortunately, therapy intervention frequently declines sharply or ceases when the child leaves the paediatric domain. In the study conducted by Bax and colleagues (1988), subjects with athetoid CP said that they had not had contractures during their school days. However, few of them had continued to take regular exercise or have physiotherapy after leaving school, and subsequently many had developed contractures and postural deformities, and some were no longer able to stand.

Of the 101 adults with CP investigated by Murphy *et al.* (1995), 64% had lower-limb contractures, rising to 91% among the non-ambulant cohort. In addition, 58 individuals had scoliosis and 15 had hip dislocation or subluxation.

Any reduction in range of movement will affect general management and prevent the attainment of an aligned and stable posture. Depending on the site and severity of these contractures, care activities such as the ability to self-feed or access the toilet may also be affected. The ability to transfer through standing or being able to walk just a few steps can significantly ease the care load (Pope 1992).

Pain

Individuals with CP do not have normal selective control of muscle activity or the anticipatory regulation of postural changes needed to protect their joints and soft-tissue structures during movement. The abrasive impact of daily life on their musculoskeletal system far exceeds that which people without disabilities experience causing impairments of the musculo-skeletal system at a young age that progress throughout adulthood and invariably give rise to pain (Gajdosik and Cicirello 2001).

Pain is therefore one of the most common secondary conditions affecting adults with CP and this increases with age (Schwartz *et al.* 1999, Gajdosik and Cicirello 2001). It may be acute or chronic and may be due to musculoskeletal deformities, arthritis or overuse syndromes. Fatigue, sustained postures, changing position after being in the same position for some time, changes in the weather, stress and depression have also been implicated as factors that exacerbate pain (Schwartz *et al.* 1999, Hodgkinson *et al.* 2001).

The physical status of a person with CP will change over time and cannot be considered as static even if movement is very limited. It is almost inevitable that the pathological movement patterns and/or sustained postures will produce abnormal stresses and strains on the musculoskeletal system leading to joint derangement and pain. Management therefore becomes a crucial issue, a key feature of any management programme being the maintenance of alignment in all positions particularly for those non-ambulant people for whom, for ex-ample, poor wheelchair seating may contribute to postural back pain (Pope 1992, Murphy *et al.* 1995).

Several studies describe an increasing incidence of pain which may be more severe in adulthood due to ageing and either disuse or overuse of muscles and limbs affected by the chronic disablement. Of 64 adults with CP, 67% reported pain in more than one site (Engel *et al.* 2002) with the lower back and legs being the most common sites (Schwartz *et al.* 1999, Turk *et al.* 2001).

It has been suggested that if patients with hip dysfunction grow up with the dysfunction untreated or inappropriately treated, the condition will continue to develop, leading to arthritis and pain in the hip (Nishioka *et al.* 2000). Cathels and Reddihough (1993) reported that there was clinical evidence of arthritis present in 27% of 66 subjects, more frequent in those who could walk, and Hodgkinson *et al.* (2001) found that hip pain was the main complaint of adults with CP with 47% of 234 non-ambulatory patients reporting hip pain.

In a study by Harada *et al.* (1993), of 84 subjects with spastic diplegia, osteoarthritis of the L5/S1 facet joints was prevalent in 67% of people over the age of 20 years with a greater than average angle of lumbar lordosis, which increased with age. In the age range 10–19 years, low back pain was a problem for 38%, this increasing to 53% in the 20–29 age range and to 64% in those over 30 years.

Although 53% of 93 subjects reported moderate to severe pain on an almost daily basis, this caused only minor interference with daily activities as a specific result of their pain. Older subjects reported higher pain intensity, a finding that may reflect the impact of ageing either through physiological changes or due to the years of muscle disuse or overuse caused by CP (Pimm 1992a, Schwartz *et al.* 1999).

Perhaps the major difficulty facing adults with CP is finding recognition that pain does not have to be accepted as an inevitable consequence of the primary condition. Hodgkinson *et al.* (2001) reported that only 13.6% of patients who complained of hip pain received medical treatment, and even then, in spite of treatment, only one was without pain. They concluded that a painful hip that does not respond to standard treatment should be referred to a pain management service.

Pain, which may result from musculoskeletal changes arising from the abnormal postures and movements, requires treatment just as it does in the able-bodied population (Edwards 2002). The musculoskeletal complaint should be acknowledged and the aetiology pursued if the pain is to be appropriately managed. Simply diagnosing 'arthritis' without considering the biomechanical factors, the ergonomics of positioning for function and the level of fitness will not direct an effective intervention programme (Turk *et al.* 2001)

Osteoporosis

Many children with CP, particularly those who are unable to walk, have decreased bone density (Flynn and Miller 2002), and a disproportionate number of adults with CP have osteoporosis that becomes worse with ageing (Rapp and Torres 2000). It is therefore not surprising that there is an increased incidence of pathological fractures in this client group. Murphy *et al.* (1995) reported that 30% of the 101 subjects in their study had a history of fractures that were thought to be attributable to disuse atrophy.

Osteoporosis related to issues of limited mobility is common in adults with CP but more research is needed to determine whether or not there is any further decrease in bone density for menopausal women with already existing secondary osteoporosis (Turk *et al.* 2001).

Increased severity of pathological movement patterns

Clinical observation suggests that the pathological movement patterns may increase in severity over time. This may be due to increased excitability due to continued use of the stereotyped patterns and/or changes in the biomechanical properties of muscle tendon complex. In both instances, the dominant muscle groups become shortened with resultant muscle imbalance between agonists and antagonists.

In severe cases, intrathecal baclofen has been used to reduce spastic hypertonia in long-standing CP. However, following this intervention, it was again emphasized that patients required rehabilitation to benefit functionally from the decreased motor tone or increased voluntary movement they experienced in order to maintain or increase range of movement and improve functional mobility (Meythaler *et al*. 2001).

Myelopathy
Cervical spondylotic myelopathy frequently occurs in association with athetoid CP, and in those who have a compensatory cervical lordosis to overcome a flexed spinal posture, and may give rise to serious secondary disability. It has been suggested that malalignment or instability of the cervical spine and osteophyte-related neural compression, secondary to cervical spondylotic changes, are the main pathological factors in the development of myelopathy (Fuji *et al*. 1987, Onari 2000, Onari *et al*. 2002). Developmental stenosis of the spinal canal has also been implicated (Fuji *et al*. 1987).

Although spondylotic changes may occur in the able-bodied population, often in the fifth decade, they usually occur earlier in people with athetoid CP, due to the persistent involuntary movements of the head and neck (Saiki *et al*. 1999). In the study by Murphy *et al*. (1995), 50% of the client group had cervical pain, increasing to 75% in those with athetoid CP.

Cervical myelopathy in people with athetoid CP may require surgery. However, various difficulties have been reported regarding stabilization of the neck post-surgery due to the involuntary neck movements that may be exacerbated by the surgical procedure. There is also a possibility of recurrence of their symptoms and therefore long-term follow-up is essential (Azuma *et al*. 2002).

Muscle-tone reducing procedures, namely partial nerve block with lignocaine and surgical release of the muscle attachment, were used prior to surgery to reduce involuntary head movements while preserving voluntary muscles forces relatively well (Saiki *et al*. 1999).

Preoperative high-dose botulinum toxin for symptomatic relief of severe dystonic neck movements has also been used in two people with dystonic CP. Side-effects of dysphagia were predicted and treated by means of a gastrostomy, and in both cases emerging respiratory complications required tracheostomy. In spite of these somewhat drastic side-effects, this intervention enabled these two patients to tolerate halofixation and allowed surgery that stopped the progression of cervical myelopathy (Racette *et al*. 1998). However, Onari *et al*. (2002) questions the long-term effectiveness of botulinum toxin on the basis that the effect would be short lasting.

Implications for ongoing management
People with CP with a significant movement disorder will require access to medical and therapy services for the rest of their lives in order to maintain their optimal level of function. As the child with CP enters the adult world, the movement disorder does not disappear with skeletal maturity; quite the contrary. As described above there are many and varied secondary conditions that will potentially lead to a progressive decrease in function. It is therefore essential to monitor this client group in order that problems can be addressed before they become irreversible.

Education
Education of all those involved in the management of this client group is essential to main-

tain optimal function. This includes those working in health, education and social services and should include greater awareness on the part of paediatric services of the long-term implications of treatment and possibly the earlier use of aids and assistive technology to reduce the stress imposed on the musculoskeletal system. With the explanation that CP is a non-progressive disorder there is often a lack of appreciation of the potential for decline on the part of the person with CP, their family and carers. This attitude may inadvertently be fostered by paediatric staff who do not have the opportunity to monitor children once they enter the adult world and therefore do not appreciate the incidence of secondary problems in adult life.

Increased emphasis is required on the identity of and the response to the changing needs of physically disabled people to maintain their optimal level of function, with improved liaison between paediatric and adult services. Coordinated adult teams would allow a planned transition from paediatric care (Cathels and Reddihough 1993), with the regular monitoring of disabled children continuing as a preventative measure throughout the course of their lifetime to prevent or delay the process of deterioration. It is recommended that a transition review should be provided regardless of whether or not children have a statement of educational need (Fiorentino *et al*. 1998).

Functional deterioration must be recognized as such by all those involved in the ongoing management of these people and not be attributed to the primary condition of CP (Williams and Bowie 1993, Murphy 1999). However, this applies not only to professional staff but also to the individuals themselves. If the person with CP and their carers do not appreciate that secondary conditions may arise, they will not make provision for physiological burnout nor will they seek help as problems emerge. This then creates a dilemma whereby unless demands are made on health, education and social services, there is unlikely to be any significant change in resources (Pimm 1992a).

Training is key to developing an ongoing management programme to enable optimal function but this must be tempered by the energy demands of accomplishing a particular task. For example, it has been suggested that the traditional approach to paediatric therapy, concentrating almost exclusively on the achievement of independent walking, may not be the ideal approach (Bottos *et al*. 2001). However, in clinical practice it is often difficult to persuade the individual with CP and their carers, that judicious use of a wheelchair may have long-term benefits in the minimization of secondary problems.

Those suffering severe and chronic neurological pathologies are a frequently neglected group in spite of an increasing survival rate (Condie 1991, Pope 1992, Bottos *et al*. 2001). While mortality is specifically linked to the severity of the condition and lack of basic functional skills namely mobility, eating/drinking and learning difficulties (Strauss and Shavelle 1998, Evans *et al*. 1990), with improved medical care, more are surviving for longer (Bottos *et al*. 2001).

The complexity of many of the secondary conditions associated with CP requires ongoing specialist consultation (Gajdosik and Cicirello 2001). Coordinated adult teams providing services similar to those in the paediatric field would allow planned transition from paediatric to adult services, which is generally recognized as being more complex for those with disability (Healy and Rigby 1999, Furukawa *et al*. 2001, Magill-Evans *et al*. 2001). This would ensure that people with physical disabilities could maintain their maximum level of functioning and independence throughout much of their lives (Cathels and Reddihough 1993).

Long-term therapy intervention

Although the terms 'management' and 'treatment' tend to be used interchangeably, they are essentially different, and it is important to make this distinction with regard to the ongoing needs of people with CP:

• *Management* is primarily concerned with "the maintenance of optimal physical condition through control of posture, movement of joints and handling techniques . . . It is primarily preventive in nature but may be corrective if secondary problems have already occurred."

• *Treatment* is "a technique or modality used or monitored by a physiotherapist for the purpose of enhancing motor performance and reducing the impairment and symptoms of the pathology" (Pope 1997).

There is obvious overlap in that appropriate management of the individual forms the basis of the attainment of optimal function, and therefore, although it is possible to have management without treatment, the reverse is not the case. An appropriate management programme should be established in childhood and should underpin all forms of therapeutic intervention. This should be carefully monitored and adapted throughout the course of the individual's lifetime. Treatment may be considered to be complementary to the underlying management and is not necessarily ongoing (Pope 1997, Edwards 2002).

Postural management should include regular standing, ongoing review of seating needs and of supports to improve the individual's position when in bed, and the provision of appropriate footwear. Hopefully, this may prevent or minimize the incidence of deformities such as hip dislocation and scoliosis that lead to significant problems with pain, seating and care-giving (Knapp and Cortes 2002). If these complications arise, the individual must be monitored throughout adult life (Gajdosik and Cicrello 2001) since, for example, for adults with CP, many relatively small curves continued to progress after skeletal maturity, the progression rate being related to the size of the curve at maturity (Majd *et al*. 1997).

The management process should include ongoing assessment to ensure continuing high-quality care for physically disabled people that remains appropriate for their needs (Williams and Bowie 1993). If a management programme is in place, this should reduce the therapy needs relating to the primary disorder of CP in the longer term. However, it will not necessarily reduce the need for specific intervention that may be required for the treatment of the secondary conditions described above.

Schoolchildren with special needs are likely to continue to have special needs when they leave school, and yet, as one mother reported, "When my child left school it was as though someone had flicked a switch" (Stevenson *et al*. 1997). If, as is frequently the case, service provision becomes fragmented for young adults with CP, greater demands are inevitably placed on the carers. It is not surprising that they have expressed anxieties about the poor provision of services and frustration in obtaining information about help. Mothers acknowledge the need to form a realistic plan for the future of their child but most of them do not know whom to turn to for help in forming such a plan (Cathels and Reddihough 1993, Stevenson *et al*. 1997).

Specific therapy programmes

It is important to promote a healthy lifestyle including participation in physical exercise, diet, developing a supportive social system and managing stress (Gajdosik and Cicirello 2001). Most individuals with disabilities are less physically active than the general population, with a relatively sedentary lifestyle, making them more susceptible to secondary health conditions (Heller *et al.* 2002). The response to exercise is similar between those with CP and the able-bodied population (Tobimatsu *et al.* 1998, Darrah *et al.* 1999), but it is essential to identify which exercises are safe and beneficial. Typical repetitive and weight-bearing activities such as running, walking and weight-lifting may need to be modified for adults with CP to preserve joint integrity (Heller *et al.* 2002).

General fitness levels are usually decreased particularly in adolescents and adults with spastic-type CP due to an increase in fat and body weight without a similar increase in muscle strength (Darrah *et al.* 1999). There is a different picture for those with dyskinetic CP where increased energy demands due to the constant athetoid movements mean they are hypermetabolic in comparison with age-matched control subjects (Johnson *et al.* 1995).

In an early study by Lundberg (1975), using a static bicycle, there was a significant difference between those with spastic and those with dyskinetic CP. This was attributed to the greater amount of energy required by the spastic group in order to overcome the constant increase in muscle tone during the test.

Darrah *et al.* (1999) conducted a 10-week community fitness programme for adults with CP who were independently mobile and reported that there was: (a) improved muscle strength; (b) no change in cardiovascular fitness (possibly because the energy demands for them to walk may already be so high that there is little room for their energy efficiency to change); (c) no significant change in flexibility; and (d) a dramatic change in their perception of their physical appearance.

It is suggested that for physical fitness to become an integral part of an individual's lifestyle, the locus of control must be within the person and not externally driven (Marge 1988 as cited by Darrah *et al.* 1999). However, it is interesting to note that when caregivers perceived greater benefits of physical exercise, adults with CP were likely to exercise more frequently (Heller *et al.* 2002).

Vogtle *et al.* (1998) reported some benefits of exercise in water in six case studies. There was improvement in the range of movement during and one month after hydrotherapy and a decrease in pain for four subjects, although three reported new sites of pain. The heart rate was unchanged. It was considered easier to bathe, dress and toilet the subjects, this being attributed to decreased stiffness and improved mobility. However, the specific aims of decreasing functional impairments and increasing social interaction were not definitely achieved.

When using specific therapy techniques for treatment of a particular secondary condition, the need for an holistic approach, utilizing specialist skills from both neurological and musculoskeletal physiotherapy, has been advocated (Tyson 1998, Plum and Morrisey 2002).

Predicting long-term therapy needs

Although the emphasis of treatment must still be on the prevention, or at least minimization of secondary complications, the outcome for adults with CP is improving with advances in medical care. With regard to life expectancy, it can be argued that, after age 30, people with CP having a more sheltered lifestyle may have a longer life expectancy than their age-matched peers. The problems encountered leading a 'normal' lifestyle with all its inherent dangers may outweigh the problems related to having CP (Miles 1995). More adults with CP are achieving competitive employment and independent living in spite of moderate to severe physical disability, and there is increasing use of improved technology such as powered wheelchairs to conserve energy for the physical demands of the job (Murphy *et al.* 2000).

Intensive treatment programmes early in life may reduce the likelihood of immobility in later life but what are the financial implications? For example, maintenance of the optimal physical condition may prevent the need for surgery, and in this way, reduce treatment costs. However, this would not necessarily lead to a reduced need for treatment in later life. CP is a condition with which one lives rather than a condition from which one dies (Evans *et al.* 1990).

When determining the cost of treatment in medico-legal cases, there is little factual information regarding the long-term therapy needs but these can be predicted based on the management issues described above. Many people with CP maintain an independent lifestyle and do not want or need regular therapy intervention. However, the danger of secondary complications remains throughout their lives: the more severe the abnormal postures, the greater the danger. Regular assessment and treatment of the secondary conditions is essential to maintain the optimal level of function (Edwards 2002).

The need for continuing services for adolescents and young adults with disabilities cannot be overemphasized (Bax 2001). Not only would monitoring and management make for a better quality of life for individuals with CP and their carers, but also in the longer term this could save the health service money, with fewer operations and admissions to hospital, and reduce the need for long-term care. This requires an appropriate handover from paediatric to adult services.

REFERENCES

Ando, N., Ueda, S. (2000) 'Functional deterioration in adults with cerebral palsy.' *Clinical Rehabilitation*, **14**, 300–306.
Andersson, C., Mattsson, E. (2001) 'Adults with cerebral palsy: a survey describing problems, needs and resources with special emphasis on locomotion.' *Developmental Medicine and Child Neurology*, **43**, 76–82.
Azuma, S., Seichi, A., Ohnishi, I., Kawaguchi, H., Kitagawa, T., Nakamura, K. (2002) 'Long-term results of operative treatment for cervical spondylotic myelopathy in patients with athetoid cerebral palsy: an over 10-year follow-up study.' *Spine*, **27**, 943–948.
Bax, M. (2001) 'Adolescence and after.' *Developmental Medicine and Child Neurology*, **43**, 435. (Editorial.)
Bax, M., Smyth, D., Thomas, A. (1988) 'Health care of physically handicapped young adults.' *British Medical Journal*, **296**, 1153–1155.
Bottos, M., Feliciangeli, A., Scuito, L., Gericke, C., Vianello, A. (2001) 'Functional status of adults with cerebral palsy and implications for treatment of children.' *Developmental Medicine and Child Neurology*, **43**, 516–528.
Cadenhead, S., McEwen, I., Thompson, D. (2002) 'Effect of passive range of motion exercises on lower-extremity goniometric measurements of adults with cerebral palsy: a single-subject design.' *Physical Therapy*, **82**, 658–669.

Cathels, B., Reddihough, D. (1993) 'The health care of young adults with cerebral palsy.' *Medical Journal of Australia*, **159**, 444–446.

Chamberlain, M.A. (1993) 'Physically handicapped school leavers.' *Archives of Disease in Childhood*, **69**, 399–402.

Condie, E. (1991) 'A therapeutic approach to physical disability.' *Physiotherapy*, **77**, 72–77.

Darrah, J., Wessel, J,. Nearingburg, P., O'Connor, M. (1999) 'Evaluation of a community fitness program for adolescents with cerebral palsy.' *Paediatric Physical Therapy*, **11**, 18–23.

Edwards, S. (2002) 'Longer-term management for patients with residual or progressive disability.' *In:* Edwards, S. (Ed.) *Neurological Physiotherapy: A Problem-Solving Approach, 2nd Edn.* London: Churchill Livingstone.

Engel, J., Kartin, D., Jensen, M. (2002) 'Pain treatment in persons with cerebral palsy: frequency and help-fulness.' *American Journal of Physical Medicine and Rehabilitation*, **81**, 291–296.

Evans, P., Evans, S., Alberman, E. (1990) 'Cerebral palsy: why we must plan for survival.' *Archives of Disease in Childhood*, **65**, 1329–1333.

Fiorentino, L., Datta, D., Gentle, S., Hall, D., Harpin, V., Phillips, D., Walker, A. (1998) 'Transition from school to adult life for physically disabled young people.' *Archives of Disease in Childhood*, **79**, 306–311.

Flynn, J., Miller, F. (2002) 'Management of hip disorders in patients with cerebral palsy.' *Journal of the American Academy of Orthopaedic Surgeons*, **10**, 198–209.

Fuji, T., Yonenobu, K., Fujiwara, K., Yamashita, K., Ebara, S., Ono, K., Okada, K. (1987) 'Cervical radiculopathy or myelopathy secondary to athetoid cerebral palsy.' *Journal of Bone and Joint Surgery, American Volume*, **69**, 815–821.

Furukawa, A., Iwatsuki, H., Nishiyama, M., Nii, E., Uchida, A. (2001) 'A study on the subjective well-being of adult patients with cerebral palsy.' *Journal of Physical Therapy Science*, **13**, 31–35.

Gajdosik, C.G., Cicirello, N. (2001) 'Secondary conditions of the musculoskeletal system in adolescents and adults with cerebral palsy.' *Physical and Occupational Therapy in Paediatrics*, **21** (4), 49–68.

Harada, T., Ebara, S., Anwar, M., Kajiura, I., Oshita, S., Hiroshima, K., Ono, K. (1993) 'The lumbar spine in spastic diplegia.' *Journal of Bone and Joint Surgery, British Volume*, **75**, 534–537.

Healy, H., Rigby, P. (1999) 'Promoting independence for teens and young adults with physical disabilities.' *Canadian Journal of Occupational Therapy*, **66**, 240–249.

Heller, T., Ying, G., Rimmer, J., Marks, B. (2002) 'Determinants of exercise in adults with cerebral palsy.' *Public Health Nursing*, **19**, 223–231.

Hodgkinson, I., Jindrich, M., Duhaut, P., Vadot, J., Metton, G., Berard, C. (2001) 'Hip pain in 234 non-ambulatory adolescents and young adults with cerebral palsy: a cross-sectional multicentre study.' *Developmental Medicine and Child Neurology*, **43**, 806–808.

Johnson, R., Goran, M., Ferrara, M., Poehlman, E. (1995) 'Athetosis increases resting metabolic rate in adults with cerebral palsy.' *Journal of the American Dietetic Association*, **95**, 145–148.

Knapp, D., Cortes, H. (2002) 'Untreated hip dislocation in cerebral palsy.' *Journal of Pediatric Orthopedics*, **22**, 668–671.

Lundberg, A. (1975) 'Mechanical effeciency in bicycle ergometer work of young adults with cerebral palsy.' *Developmental Medicine and Child Neurology*, **17**, 434–439.

Magill-Evans, J., Darrah, J., Pain, K., Adkins, R., Kratochvil, M. (2001) 'Are families with adolescents and young adults with cerebral palsy the same as other families?' *Developmental Medicine and Child Neurology*, **43**, 466–472.

Majd, M.E., Muldowny, D.S., Holt, R.T. (1997) 'Natural history of scoliosis in the institutionalized adult cerebral palsy population.' *Spine*, **22**, 1461–1466.

Mayston, M. (2001) 'People with cerebral palsy: effects of and perspectives for therapy.' *Neural Plasticity*, **8**, 51–69.

Meythaler, J., Guin-Renfroe, S., Law, C., Grabb, P., Hadley, M. (2001) 'Continuously infused intrathecal baclofen over 12 months for spastic hypertonia in adolescents and adults with cerebral palsy.' *Archives of Physical Medicine and Rehabilitation*, **82**, 155–161.

Miles, R. (1995) 'Life expectancy in cerebral palsy.' *Developmental Medicine and Child Neurology*, **37**, 1115. (Letter.)

Murphy, K. (1999) 'Medical problems in adults with cerebral palsy: case examples.' *Assistive Technology*, **11**, 97–104.

Murphy, K., Molnar, G., Lankasky, K. (1995) 'Medical and functional status of adults with cerebral palsy.' *Developmental Medicine and Child Neurology*, **37**, 1075–1084.

Murphy, K., Molnar, G., Lankasky, K. (2000) 'Employment and social issues in adults with cerebral palsy.' *Archives of Physical Medicine and Rehabilitation*, **81**, 807–811.

Nishioka, E., Momota, K., Shiba, N., Higuchi, F., Inoue, A. (2000) 'Joint-preserving operation for osteoarthrosis of the hip in adult cerebral palsy.' *Australian and New Zealand Journal of Surgery*, **70**, 431–437.

Onari, K. (2000) 'Surgical treatment for cervical spondylotic myelopathy associated with cerebral palsy.' *Journal of Orthopaedic Science*, **5**, 439–448.

Onari, K., Kondo, S., Mihara, H., Iwamira, Y. (2002) 'Combined anterior–posterior fusion for cervical spondylotic myelopathy in patients with athetoid cerebral palsy.' *Journal of Neuroscience*, **97**, 13–19.

Pimm, P. (1992a) 'Cerebral palsy: a non-progressive disorder?' *Educational and Child Psychology*, **9**, 27–33.

Pimm, P. (1992b) 'Physiological burn-out and functional skill loss in cerebral palsy.' *Interlink*, **4** (3), 18–20.

Pimm, P. (1996) 'Some of the implications of caring for a child or adult with cerebral palsy.' *British Journal of Occupational Therapy*, **59**, 335–341.

Plum, H., Morrissey, D. (2002) 'Cross speciality collaboration.' *Physiotherapy*, **88**, 530–533.

Pope, P. (1992) 'Management of the physical condition in patients with chronic and severe neurological pathologies.' *Physiotherapy*, **78**, 896–903.

Pope, P. (1997) 'Management of the physical condition in people with chronic and severe neurological disabilities living in the community.' *Physiotherapy*, **83**, 116–122.

Racette, B., Lauryssen, C., Perlmutter, J. (1998) 'Preoperative treatment with botulinum toxin to facilitate cervical fusion in dystonic cerebral palsy.' *Journal of Neurosurgery*, **88**, 328–330.

Rapp, C., Torres, M. (2000) 'The adult with cerebral palsy.' *Archives of Family Medicine*, **9**, 466–472.

Saiki, K., Tsuzuki, N., Tanaka, R. (1999) 'The effect of muscle tone reducing procedures in athetotic head movements: partial nerve block by lidicaine and surgical release of the neck muscles.' *Clinical Neurophysiology*, **110**, 1308–1314.

Schwartz, L., Engel, J., Jensen, M. (1999) 'Pain in persons with cerebral palsy.' *Archives of Physical Medicine and Rehabilitation*, **80**, 1243–1246.

Stevenson, C., Pharoah, P., Stevenson, R. (1997) 'Cerebral palsy—the transition from youth to adulthood.' *Developmental Medicine and Child Neurology*, **39**, 336–342.

Strauss, D., Shavelle, R. (1998) 'Life expectancy of adults with cerebral palsy.' *Developmental Medicine and Child Neurology*, **40**, 369–375.

Tardieu, C., Lespargot, A., Tabary, C., Bret, M.D. (1988) 'For how long must the soleus muscle be stretched each day to prevent contracture?' *Developmental Medicine and Child Neurology*, **30**, 3–10.

Tobimatsu, Y., Nakamura, R., Kusano, S., Iwasaki, Y. (1998) 'Cardiorespiratory endurance in people with cerebral palsy measured using an arm ergometer.' *Archives of Physical Medicine and Rehabilitation*, **79**, 991–993.

Turk, M.A., Scandale, J., Rosenbaum, P.F., Weber, R.J. (2001) 'The health of women with cerebral palsy.' *Physical Medicine and Rehabilitation Clinics of North America*, **12**, 153–168.

Tyson, S. (1998) 'The use of musculoskeletal techniques in adult cerebral palsy.' *Physiotherapy Research International*, **3**, 292–295.

van der Dussen, L., Nieuwstraten, W., Roebroeck, M., Stam, H.J. (2001) 'Functional level of young adults with cerebral palsy.' *Clinical Rehabilitation*, **15**, 84–91.

Vogtle, L., Morris, D., Denton, B. (1998) 'An aquatic programme for adults with cerebral palsy living in group homes.' *Physical Therapy Case Reports*, **1**, 250–259.

Williams, M., Bowie, C. (1993) 'Evidence of unmet need in the care of severely disabled adults.' *British Medical Journal*, **306**, 95–98.

13
THERAPEUTIC POSSIBILITIES: RESEARCH OVERVIEW AND COMMENTARY

Murray Goldstein

By definition, cerebral palsy (CP) is a non-progressive disorder of the developing brain that expresses itself early in infancy and childhood as impaired function of neuromuscular control. It is a syndrome characterized by multiple aetiologies, a variety of pathologies, several motor control deficits and a number of comorbidities. Common coexisting nervous system problems include visual impairment, hearing loss, cognitive difficulties, behavioural disturbances and convulsive disorders. Improved quality of life is a universal goal of all persons with disabilities due to CP. The achievement of that goal involves the collaborative activity of persons with CP, families, caregivers, clinicians, scientists and the community. Within that goal, a major health objective is the elimination or lessening of the impairments (*e.g.* muscle spasticity, involuntary movements) and the disabilities (*e.g.* mobility restriction, limited communication skills) identified with CP. It is a difficult objective to achieve because of the still incomplete knowledge about the one or more injuries to the developing brain that are the basis of motor impairment and functional disability. However, important progress has already been made for the lessening of impairment, the improvement of function and the development of community programmes for improved clinical and societal services. In addition, progress is being made steadily for the better management of disabilities as more is learned about the injured brain and the neuromuscular coordination systems it controls. Important also is the recognition that persons with CP often have a broad spectrum of coexisting disorders that need appropriate attention. Future progress is dependant both upon advances in biological and clinical knowledge and equally on the improvement and availability of clinical, family and community resources to use that knowledge effectively.

Treating the injured brain
As of this time, there are no clinically meaningful interventions that are able to successfully *repair* the focal damage done to the motor system of the developing brain. Implantation of embryonic and fetal cells into selected areas of the injured brain has been studied in adult-onset disorders to enhance the environment for the repair of damaged neural cells and to replace destroyed cells (Snyder *et al.* 1997, Bjorklund *et al.* 2002, Ourednik *et al.* 2002, Park *et al.* 2002). This has been done in both animal and human studies of Parkinson's disease and in cerebral infarction secondary to cerebral ischaemia. In Parkinson's disease, there has been transient improvement in motor function following implantation of embryonic cells into the basal ganglia, but with only a relatively short-term beneficial effect on function. In stroke, there has also been a very short-lived positive result. The efficacy of the implantation

in brain of more primitive, omnipotential stem cells is now under investigation. Parkinson's disease and cerebral infarction have again been the models of focal brain injury that have been used. Again, positive results have been minimal, but in younger Parkinson's disease patients the undesirable side-effect of dyskenesia has occurred. Research on the implantation of stem cells continues in animal models, including young animals with experimental brain injury. A recent finding indicates that in addition to the potential for reestablishing the integrity of injured neuronal networks and establishing new neuronal networks, stem cells appear to be able to release neurotrophic factors that assist in adjacent brain cell repair and growth. Although stem cell research continues to offer promise for repair of the damage due to focal brain injury with a resulting improvement in function, to date the beneficial effects are very limited and the clinical potential remains guarded.

Another approach to restoring brain function due to developmental brain injury is that of mobilizing the biological phenomenon known as brain *plasticity* in order to recruit other areas of brain—often adjacent areas—to perform functions that have been lost due to focal injury. The microstructural and biochemical anatomy of the developing and mature brain is constantly changing in response to alterations in their environment. These changes are the biological basis of learning. As a result, the brain is able to acquire new motor control abilities and improve upon existing motor performance. The important role of sensory system input to enhance plasticity has recently been emphasized. These studies indicate that interventions using targeted sensory input coupled with structured motor demand can bring about subtle changes in brain synapse configuration resulting in improved motor performance (Nudo *et al.* 1996). One example of this is the positive results reported for the use of 'constraint-induced therapy' to improve functional performance of the impaired limb in hemiplegia (Taub *et al.* 1993). The resulting functional changes are often transient initially, but with repetition can become long lasting. Also, techniques of 'programmed learning' leading to changes in brain structure (synapse formation and/or activation) have been demonstrated to improve motor performance. In animal models, it has been reported that motor performance can be further enhanced by the concurrent use of stimulatory drugs such as amphetamine; this is presently under study in adult humans with hempleia following cerebral infarction.

Another approach has been the introduction of neurotrophic agents into the area of injury to enhance the recovery of injured but viable cells and to encourage the recruitment of adjacent cells to participate in motor activity. These agents have usually been hormonal in nature, but recently stem cell metabolites have been utilized. Again, there appear to be modest positive results as measured by the impact on impairment. However, the function that has been restored or improved upon has often been modest and is sometimes associated with unde-sirable associated involuntary movements. It has been suggested that the mobilization of alternative neuronal pathways may improve gross performance; however, they have been found to be less specific or efficient than the primary pathways. The role of brain plasticity in restoring meaningful function lost by developmental brain injury is an increasingly active area of scientific investigation; specifically, studies are underway to identify which motor areas of brain are most susceptible to plastic changes of importance and what stimuli are needed to enhance changes in the brain of functional significance.

In summary, research in animal models of brain injury demonstrate that partial repair of focal areas of the injured brain by implantation of primitive cells is possible; also that by means of targeted stimuli and repetition, permanent changes can be brought about in brain via synapse reconfiguration and activation (plasticity). Under experimental conditions in animal models, each of these approaches has resulted in modest improvements in motor performance. Minimal adverse effects can occur but have been clinically manageable. In observational and experimental studies of humans with deficits in motor performance, clinically meaningful results to date are limited. However, the possibility now exists that the injured human brain can be partially repaired or restructured with resulting improvement in performance.

In addition to the above-mentioned conventional scientific approaches to brain-injury repair and enhanced plasticity, over time a host of *complementary and alternative medical (CAM) approaches* have been proposed as interventions to repair damaged brain and restore lost function. Some of the CAM approaches for improving brain function are dietary supplements, herbal extracts, electrical and magnetic brain stimulation, acupuncture, patterning, craniosacral manipulation, force-field therapy, and hyperbaric oxygen administration. People with disabilities and their caregivers have turned to these unconventional interventions because of their dissatisfaction with the results of conventional therapies and their impatience with the uncertainty of clinically relevant results of scientific investigations of brain repair or remodeling. Reports of the success of CAM approaches are often anecdotal in character and are usually provided by CAM participants, both clinical care practitioners and patients or their caregivers. However, *controlled clinical evaluations are usually lacking*, particularly evaluations that include the now accepted principles underlying the use of the clinical trial methodologies: specified criteria for subject inclusion and exclusion, predetermined and measurable end-points, short- and long-term follow-ups, blinded evaluation and the use of controls (Butler *et al.* 1999). Clinical experience and family evaluation are usually offered as the evidence in support of CAM therapies. However, it is now generally accepted that in human-oriented research, clinical experience and family observations are fertile fields for hypothesis formulation, but are rarely adequate as evidence in support of an hypothesis.

Another issue in the evaluation of most CAM approaches to therapy is 'proof of principle', namely evidence of a demonstrated biological basis in support of the clinical observation. A biological explanation of a change in structure or/and function is usually required to justify the investment of the substantial resources necessary to investigate a specific experimental or innovative intervention. Theoretical explanations of biological change are often offered as the basis for CAM approaches used for interventions to ameliorate disabilities associated with CP; however, scientifically acceptable evidence of the validity of these biological suppositions is nearly always lacking.

One exception to the lack of meaningful information obtained from controlled clinical trials of CAM procedures is a recently reported randomized clinical trial of hyperbaric oxygen therapy (HBOT) administered to children with spastic diplegia associated with CP (Collet *et al.* 2001). The investigators found that air administered at 1.3 ata (a 'placebo') provided the same clinical results as did 100% oxygen administered at 1.7 ata. They concluded that HBOT was no more effective than the placebo and suggested that participation in a clinical trial in itself could lead to limited degrees of improved performance. Advocates of HBOT dispute the study conclusion that hyperbaric oxygen was not efficacious. They point out that hyperbaric air administered at very low levels of hyperbaria (1.3 ata) provides for an increased oxygen saturation of blood equivalent to inhalation of 25% oxygen by face mask. They suggest, instead, that the trial demonstrates that even modest levels of HBOT are clinically efficacious. There has been no direct scientific response to this suggestion, but existing biologic data indicate that very modest increases in oxygen saturation of blood (*e.g.* 25% oxygen administered by face mask) have not been shown to have a physiological effect on brain cell metabolism.

Another issue in considering the efficacy of HBOT is a lack of proof of principle. HBOT advocates hypothesize that four to eight years after brain injury children still have 'resting brain cells' in the area of injury (penumbra?) that can be 'activated' by HBOT to become functional. There is no meaningful evidence at this time in support of that hypothesis. This lack of acceptable evidence recognizes that SPECT scans demonstrate in some subjects an increase of regional blood flow following HBOT therapy. However, regional blood flow increase is not synonymous with an increase in focal brain cell metabolism. Studies in other paradigms such as cerebral infarction due to hypoxia–ischaemia indicate that a penumbra (the presence of brain cells at the margins of an infarction that function at a low metabolic rate) is a short-lived phenomenon and is present for only hours after the insult, not for years. Metabolic studies demonstrating a focal increase in cerebral metabolism as measured by PET scans would be necessary to test the 'resting brain cells' hypothesis.

Since the brain injury resulting in CP can be due to a host of very different aetiologies (*e.g.* migratory cell disturbance, poor myelination of axons and dendrites, neuronal cell loss, synaptic dysfunction, etc.), the effectiveness of a single intervention such as HBOT repairing a host of different pathologies seems improbable. Perhaps future studies may show a beneficial effect of HBOT in selected circumstances. However, at this time there is no biologically or clinically acceptable evidence to support the use of HBOT for the treatment of the brain injury resulting in CP or in the management of the motor impairments and disabilities resulting from that injury.

In summary, experience shows that CAM therapies for CP such as HBOT are introduced regularly, gain popularity in a relatively small advocacy group of clinicians and patients (often parents of young patients), are vigorously promoted by the advocacy group, usually remain unevaluated by scientifically reliable studies, and then after several years generally lose popularity as the long-term results fail to justify their often high cost in time commitment and funds. Nevertheless, clinicians and scientists must remain open-minded and consider the evidence in support of each CAM approach individually because experience also demonstrates that unconventional interventions are sometimes proven to be efficacious and are then incorporated into conventional clinical practice. It must also be acknowledged that a large proportion of interventions presently used in conventional therapy of developmental brain injury and its consequences are supported only by years of experience and like CAM have not been subjected to scientifically vigorous studies of either proof of principle or clinical efficacy.

Management of functional loss in the neuromuscular coordination system and of impairments of skeletal alignment

Developmental brain injury manifests itself functionally in a variety of ways including sensory and motor disturbances, cognitive loss, behavioural perturbations and convulsive disorders. Although the several different brain injuries resulting in CP are at the upper motor neuron level, the principal clinical manifestation is an impairment of motor coordination at the lower motor neuron level. The final common pathway of functional disturbance in CP is in the neuromuscular coordination system at levels of the spinal cord and peripheral nerve. Muscle spasticity, muscle weakness, poor muscle coordination and/or involuntary movements are the usual manifestations of that disturbance. Thus, clinical interventions to modulate these impairments and improve function are aimed at the way stations of the neuromuscular coordination system. At the spinal cord level, GABA agonists (*e.g.* baclofen) have been used intrathecally and have successfully diminished peripheral sensory and motor nerve hyperexcitability (Butler and Campbell 2000, Albright *et al.* 2001). At the neuromuscular junction, focal synaptic transmission has been interrupted successfully by the local administration of botulinum toxin (*e.g.* BTX-A). Neurosurgical sectioning of afferent neurons at the paraspinal region (dorsal rhizotomy) has also been used successfully to diminish sensory input into the spinal cord (McLaughlin *et al.* 1998). Finally, a host of mood elevating and muscle relaxant oral medications have been used with modest results to lessen overall sensitivity to environmental stimuli.

When used selectively and skillfully, each of these interventions has been demonstrated clinically to be successful in diminishing impairment, primarily muscle spasticity. This has usually led to improved personal hygiene, better body positioning and improved self-image; all are important therapeutic objectives. However, the evidence that they concurrently lead to improved function *per se* is as yet fragmentary. The modulation or elimination of a pathophysiological impairment does not equate with an improvement of function. Following pharmacologic or surgical intervention, the clinical care responsibility for improvement of function has often been that of clinical therapists in the disciplines of physiotherapy, occupational therapy, behavioral therapy, speech therapy and special education.

Improved function leading to independence and the ability to better participate in personal, family and community activities is a key goal of all clinical interventions for persons with disabilities, including those due to CP. The clinical therapist is usually identified with the responsibility of assisting the person with a disability both to improve function and to maintain existing function over time. Approaches used usually include establishment of therapeutic goals, relaxation of spastic muscles, strengthening of weak muscles, improving muscle coordination, and enhancing motivation and ability to participate in activities of daily living. A host of methodologies have been developed in each discipline to accomplish these objectives. The different methodologies all appear to have positive results. Their success appears to be dependent upon the skill and enthusiasm of the therapist and the motivation and cooperation of the subject rather than on the specifics of the therapeutic methodology. Protocol-based studies utilizing controls are just being initiated to evaluate the comparative efficacy of the individual 'schools of therapy' under specified circumstances; the variables that are considered include type and duration of disability, age of the subject, comorbidities and characteristics of the environment (Law *et al*. 1997, Bower *et al*. 2001, Trahan and Malouin 2002). Also, quantitative methodologies measuring performance (Sutherland *et al*. 1996) and qualitative scales of activity (Russell *et al*. 2002) are becoming available to evaluate efficacy in these studies. At the present time, however, the choice of which therapy to use is usually made on the basis of the educational background of the clinical therapist and their clinical impression of its efficacy.

One of the results of the present lack of meaningful data is the regular introduction of a new or different 'school of therapy'. Characteristic of the successful school are the dynamic interaction of its founder(s) with students of that school and the therapist's supportive interaction with the person receiving therapy and their family. The observation that each of these therapeutic systems seems to work when utilized by a skilled and sensitive practitioner lends support to the supposition that the important variables may be the increased motivation and involvement of the subject rather than the specifics of the intervention itself. However, that remains to be evaluated.

Four important and as yet unanswered questions in all methodologies ('schools') of clinical therapy are: for whom? when? how much? and for how long? Also, what are the personal and societal factors that should determine timing, intensity and duration of therapy? In many societies, these are determined by availability and economic factors rather than clinical evidence. Also, a significant improvement in present performance is usually used as the compelling endpoint by funding sources; therapy to maintain present performance is rarely considered by them to be an important objective. Each of these issues demands attention. In order to accomplish this, additional clinical therapists need to develop the research skills necessary to investigate these questions, and research funding sources need to recognize the priority attention they deserve. Without additional research, it is easy to predict that clinical impression and patient perception of, and availability of financial support for therapy will continue to be the criteria governing the selection and use of clinical therapies to improve function for persons with disabilities.

Therapeutic electrical stimulation (TES) has been suggested as an adjunct to physiotherapy to improve motor performance. This technique, utilizing low-intensity, long-duration electrical stimulation to the skin overlying a weak muscle appears to be able to maintain and sometimes increase the mass of that muscle. Several trials of incorporating TES into home programmes of physiotherapy have provided data in support of only modest (if any) improvement in motor performance (Hazlewood 1994, Sommerfelt *et al*. 2001). However, patients resist long-term use of the methodology, and in most instances performance over time reverts to that which can be expected with physiotherapy or exercise alone.

Finally, orthopaedic surgery and orthotic devices are now available to address skeletal structural misalignments and joint fixations that are due to muscle spasticity, tendon fibrosis and contractures. The most common surgical procedures are tendon lengthening or release, tendon transfer and osteotomy. These procedures clearly achieve their anatomical alignment objective. In a few situations, the anatomical realignment in itself restores function. However, in most situations, the procedure sets the anatomic stage for other clinical procedures such as physiotherapy to address functional improvement. Fixed and dynamic othotic devices are aids to assist in accomplishing this therapeutic goal in selected clinical situations. A number of controlled clinical trials have demonstrated that the use of casting with BTX-A and physiotherapy provides for minimally better functional outcomes as compared to the same regimen without the use of BTX-A (Sutherland and Kaufman 1999).

In summary, medications and surgical procedures have been demonstrated in controlled studies to be efficacious for the control or elimination of muscle spasticity. However, they do not of themselves improve function. Instead they provide a biological environment in which techniques used by clinical therapists seek to improve and maintain muscle strength and coordination and diminish disability.

Surgical procedures and orthotic devices are available to improve skeletal alignment and joint mobility. However, the efficacy of each of these interventions is usually based on clinical observations and/or gait analysis. Most are accepted procedures in conventional medical care, but with rare exception the criteria for their use and the reports of their efficacy are based upon the experience of the highly skilled clinicians using them.

At this time, there are two schools of unconventional physical therapy receiving increasing attention by parents of children with moderate to severe disabilities due to CP: Conductive Education (Coleman *et al.* 1995, Reddihough *et al.* 1998) and a Russian–Polish rehabilitation programme incorporating the use of the Adeli suit (Semanova 1997). Both share a common feature: each originated in Eastern European cultures in which relatively lengthy and intense immersions in physiotherapy are common (*e.g.* 6–8 hours per day of a structured programme of therapy for at least one month). Recent studies comparing the Conductive Education methodology with a more conventional methodology indicate that when both are administered with the same intensity (hours/day) and duration (number of consecutive days), the results as measured by improved performance are the same; subjects randomized to each therapy both have similar improvements in performance. Again, the important questions in every school of physical therapy, conventional or CAM, appear to be: for whom? when? how much? how long? and not, what type? In regard to the Adeli suit, carefully designed studies are now in progress to evaluate its contribution to body and limb control when used in a conventional physiotherapy programme and in the Russian–Polish methodology of physiotherapy. These studies should provide the information needed to evaluate the role of this device in providing for better body stability and improved limb control.

Ageing with a developmental disability
Children with a developmental disability become adults with a developmental disability. Because of personal and societal factors, adults with a disability often can now have a full or nearly full life span and become 'aged'. Are persons with disabilities due to CP more susceptible to the dysfunctions usually associated with ageing than are the general population? There are surprisingly few reliable data available to answer that question.

Although the area(s) of focal brain injury in persons with CP are believed not to change significantly over time, the disabilities resulting from that injury are changing on a continuing basis. Each disability can remain the same, get better or get worse due to a variety of biological and environmental factors. However, ageing persons often develop a host of health problems over time that impact on well-being; this is true irrespective of the presence of a developmental disability. Some of these problems are: joint pain, muscle weakness, fatigue,

189

obesity, constipation, urinary incontinence, gastric reflux, pulmonary insufficiency, cardio-vascular disease and forgetfulness. Is the person with a developmental disability more at risk of these health problems than are others? No one knows. It is said they are; it is also said that these problems occur earlier in the ageing process in persons with developmental disabilities than in the general population. Again, no one knows. With very rare exceptions, there have been no controlled studies of the long-term health status of persons with develop-mental disabilities. Obviously, until studies are done addressing these questions, we will continue to have to guess at their answers relying on experience and case reports.

Conclusion

Reliable information about the possible treatment of the injured brain of persons with CP is beginning to indicate that some repair of the injured brain is an attainable goal. Clinical interventions for the better management of impairments and disabilities associated with CP are being developed and evaluated using controlled clinical trial methodologies. However, most clinical interventions used at this time, conventional and CAM, are based on clinical experience rather than on the results of scientific investigations. As in the past, some persons with developmental disabilities and their families who are dissatisfied with the results of conventional therapies turn to CAM approaches. Both conventional interventions and CAM therapies need to be studied for proof of principle and evaluated for efficacy using controlled clinical trial methodologies. Until this happens, persons with disabilities due to CP will have to continue to rely almost exclusively on their confidence in their clinicians and the therapeutic interventions available at the time; also, clinicians will continue to be dependent upon the teachings of their professional leaders rather than on the products of evidence-based clinical care studies. Fortunately, programmes are now in place to recruit and prepare clinician-investigators to address these questions of health care significance and to fund their research.

"If you think research is expensive, try ignorance" — Derek Bok.

REFERENCES

Albright, A.L., Barry, M.J., Shafton, D.H., Ferson, S.S. (2001) 'Intrathecal baclofen for generalized dsystonia.' *Developmental Medicine and Child Neurology*, **43**, 652–657.

Bower, E., Michell, D., Burnett, M., Campbell, M.J., McLellan, D.L. (2001) 'Randomized controlled trial of physiotherapy in 56 children with cerebral palsy followed for 18 months.' *Developmental Medicine and Child Neurology*, **43**, 4–15.

Bjorklund, L.M., Sanchez-Pernaute, R., Chung, S., Andersson, T., Chen, I.Y., McNaught, K.S., Brownell, A.L., Jenkins, B.G., Wahlestedt, C., Kim, K.S., Isacson, O. (2002) 'Embryonic stem cells develop into functional dopaminergic neurons after transplantation in a Parkinson rat model.' *Proceedings of the National Academy of Sciences of the USA*, **99**, 2344–2349.

Butler, C., Chambers, H., Goldstein, M., Harris, S., Leach, J., Campbell, S., Adams, R., Darrah, J. (1999) 'Evaluating research in developmental disabilities: a conceptual framework for reviewing treatment outcomes.' *Developmental Medicine and Child Neurology*, **41**, 55–59.

Butler, C., Campbell, S. (2000) 'Evidence of the effects of intrathecal baclofen for spastic and dystonic cerebral palsy.' Developmental Medicine and Child Neurology, 42, 634–645.

Coleman, G.J., King, J.A., Reddihough, D.S. (1995) 'A pilot evaluation of conductive education-based inter-vention for children with cerebral palsy: the Tongala Project.' *Journal of Paediatrics and Child Health*, **31**, 412–417.

Collet, J.P., Vanasse, M., Marois, P., Amar, M., Goldberg, J., Lambert, J., Lassonde, M., Hardy, P., Fortin, J., Tremblay, S.D., Montgomery, D., Lacroix, J., Robinson, A., Majnemer, A. (2001) 'Hyperbaric oxygen for children with cerebral palsy: a randomised multicentre trial. HBO-CP Research Group.' *Lancet*, **357**, 582–586.

Hazlewood, M.E., Brown, J.K., Rowe, P.J., Salter, P.M. (1994) 'The use of therapeutic electrical stimulation in the treatment of hemiplegic cerebral palsy.' *Developmental Medicine and Child Neurology*, **36**, 661–673.

Law, M., Russell, D., Pollock, N., Rosenbaum, P., Walter, S., King, G. (1997) 'A comparison of intensive neurodevelopmental therapy plus casting and a regular occupational therapy program for children with cerebral palsy.' *Developmental Medicine and Child Neurology*, **39**, 664–670.

McLaughlin, J.F., Bjornson, K.F., Astley, S.J., Graubert, C., Hays, R.M., Roberts, T.S., Price, R., Temkin, N. (1998) 'Selective dorsal rhizotomy: efficacy and safety in an investigator-masked randomized clinical trial.' *Developmental Medicine and Child Neurology*, **40**, 220–232.

Nudo, R.J., Wise, B.M., SiFuentes, F., Milliken, G.W. (1996) 'Neural substrates for the effects of rehabilitative training on motor recovery after ischemic infarct.' *Science*, **272**, 1791–1794.

Ourednik, J., Ourednik, V., Lynch, W.P., Schachner, M., Snyder, E.Y. (2002) 'Neural stem cells display an inherent mechanism for rescuing dysfunctional neurons.' *Nature Biotechnology*, **20**, 1103–1110.

Park, K.I., Teng, Y.D., Snyder, E.Y. (2002) 'The injured brain interacts reciprocally with neural stem cells supported by scaffolds to reconstitute lost tissue.' *Nature Biotechnology*, **20**, 1111–1117.

Reddihough, D.S., King, J., Coleman, G., Catanese ,T. (1998) 'Efficacy of programmes based on Conductive Education for young children with cerebral palsy.' *Developmental Medicine and Child Neurology*, **40**, 763–770.

Russell, D.J., Rosenbaum, P.L., Avery, L.M., Lane, M. (2002) *Gross Motor Function Measure (GMFM-66 and GMFM-88) User's Manual. Clinics in Developmental Medicine No. 159.* London: Mac Keith Press.

Semanova, K.A. (1997) 'Basis for a method of dynamic proprioceptive correction in the restorative treatment of patients with residual-stage infantile cerebral palsy.' *Neuroscience and Behavioral Physiology*, **27**, 639–643.

Snyder, E.Y., Yoon, C., Flax, J.D., Macklis, J.D. (1997) 'Multipotent neural precursors can differentiate toward replacement of neurones undergoing targeted apoptotic degeneration in adult mouse neocortex.' *Proceedings of the National Academy of Sciences of the USA*, **94**, 11663–11668.

Sommerfelt, K., Markestad, T., Berg, K., Saetesdal, I. (2001) 'Therapeutic electrical stimulation in cerebral palsy: a randomized, controlled, crossover trial.' *Developmental Medicine and Child Neurology*, **43**, 609–613.

Sutherland, D.H., Kaufman, K.R. (1996) 'Human motion analysis and pediatric orthopedics.' *In:* Harris, G.F., Smith, P.A. (Eds.) *Human Motion Analysis, Current Applications and Future Directions.* Piscataway, NJ: IEEE Press, pp. 219–254.

Sutherland, D.H., Kaufman, K.R., Wyatt, M.P., Chambers, H.G., Mubarak, S.J. (1999) 'Double-blind study of botulinum A toxin injections into the gastrocnemius muscle in patients with cerebral palsy.' *Gait and Posture*, **10**, 1–9.

Taub, E., Miller, N.E., Novack, T.A., Cook, E.W., Fleming, W.C., Nepomuceno, C.S., Connell, J.S., Crago, J.E. (1993) 'Technique to improve chronic motor deficit after stroke.' *Archives of Physical Medicine and Rehabilitation*, **74**, 347–354.

Trahan, J., Malouin, F. (2002) 'Intermittent intensive physiotherapy in children with cerebral palsy: a pilot study.' *Developmental Medicine and Child Neurology*, **44**, 233–239.

INDEX

195